Twenty-First Century Plague

Twenty-First Century Plague
THE STORY OF SARS

Thomas Abraham

The Johns Hopkins University Press
Baltimore, Maryland

First published in 2004 by Hong Kong University Press
Hardcover edition first published in the United States in 2005
by the Johns Hopkins University Press under license from
Hong Kong University Press, the University of Hong Kong,
Pok Fu Lam Road, Hong Kong

Johns Hopkins paperback edition 2007
9 8 7 6 5 4 3 2 1

The Johns Hopkins University Press
2715 North Charles Street
Baltimore, Maryland 21218–4363
www.press.jhu.edu

ISBN 10: 0-8018-8632-5
ISBN 13: 978-0-8018-8632-4

Library of Congress Control Number: 2004110230

A catalog record for this book is available from the British Library.

CONTENTS

PREFACE

IN the last week of April 2006, a 37-year-old woman and her extended family sat down to a feast in the village of Kubu Sembelang in the lush Karo highlands of north Sumatra in Indonesia. There is some confusion about what they ate that day; some accounts say it was a pig that was barbecued. Others say they ate chicken. The Karo people, the indigenous inhabitants of the volcanic northern Sumatra plateau, are a close-knit community, and it is difficult for outsiders to get precise information about an incident that has brought notoriety and unwelcome publicity to the village. But the details are not important. Perhaps what is more important is that a few days later, the woman, Puji Ginting, fell ill with a high fever and a cough that came from deep in her lungs. One by one, other members of her family succumbed. In the first two weeks of May, her two sons, 19-year-old Roy Karo-karo and 18-year-old Boni, her sister Anta Boru Ginting, her 8-year-old nephew Rafael, and her one-and-a-half-year-old niece Brenata and her brother all died after being admitted to hospital with high fevers and infected lungs.

Their deaths brought the numbers of human cases in Indonesia of H5N1 avian influenza to 40 since the outbreak began in 2003. But what caused greater than normal alarm was the possibility that this time the virus had not passed to the victims from infected birds, but rather from another human being.

Health officials from the Indonesian government in Jakarta, as well as scientists from the World Health Organization, descended on Kubu Sembelang village, collecting samples from hens, pigs, and people, searching for clues to how the family had caught the virus. Did they keep chicken or pigs? Had the infected family been in close contact with other villagers? Had any other villagers fallen ill? Virus samples from the ill family were sent to laboratories in Hong Kong and the US for genetic testing. Local and international news organizations arrived at the scene and local television broadcast footage of the unfortunate family in hospital.

SARS too had started like this: with individuals and then small groups of people in small towns falling ill from a disease that doctors did not know how to cure. SARS broke out in the small towns of Guangdong province in southern China, and no one in the outside world knew of its existence until nearly four months after the outbreak began. Even then, details of what had happened and the extent of the disease were sketchy.

It was because of SARS that the deaths in a village like Kubu Sembilang had come to be seen as events that deserved global attention. SARS made people acutely aware of the awful human and economic toll that infectious disease could exact from the modern world. While scientists had been warning of the possibility of a new influenza pandemic for years, few took it seriously until SARS came along in 2003.

SARS took the world by surprise. The virus that caused it was previously unknown to science, and in the first weeks after it exploded onto the world, scientists and doctors struggled to make sense of this new disease. They had never come across a respiratory virus that was seemingly resistant to anti-viral drugs, caused such severe damage to lungs, and was passed so easily and with such lethal effect from patients to the doctors and nurses who were trying to fight the disease.

No disease had ever had such an immediate global impact. After incubating and spreading in southern China, aided by a policy of official denials, the disease erupted onto the outside world through Hong Kong. The speed of modern airline travel allowed the virus to be carried by infected travellers to Singapore and Vietnam in hours and to Canada in less than a day. Besides the human costs of the disease, the economic costs were also enormous. People stopped travelling to SARS affected areas, and airports, airlines, hotels, and the travel industry felt the pinch. Factories and offices shut down as employees felt reluctant to risk going to work and falling ill.

SARS was a relatively short epidemic. The first cases arose in China in November 2002, and the last case was reported in Taiwan in June 2003. By early July the World Health Organization was able to declare that the epidemic had been contained world wide. But this was enough to give the world a taste of what an infectious disease epidemic caused by a new virus could be like. It was the perfect dress rehearsal for an influenza pandemic.

SARS forced governments to take the risk of infectious disease epidemics far more seriously than they otherwise would have. Despite the rapid increase over the last few decades of infectious diseases caused by previously unknown viruses, protecting societies against these diseases was not seen as a major priority for governments. HIV/AIDS was the only one of these new diseases that had become a global priority, but even then it took a decade or two after the disease's emergence for the world to take it seriously. Because of the SARS experience, governments have begun to see the need to prepare for pandemic influenza and to devote resources to stockpiling drugs and stimulating research into vaccines.

In the cities and region that were affected, SARS was a perfect dress rehearsal for an influenza pandemic. Health workers and hospital systems experienced the pressures, panics, and fears of coping with a seemingly endless flow of desperately ill patients. Health administrators realized how critical it was to have enough intensive care beds in hospitals. Governments were made aware of the extraordinary political and administrative demands of coping with disease. For the countries that escaped SARS, the successes and failures of the countries that experienced it are a valuable source of information on what to expect.

While we are alert to the dangers of an influenza pandemic, global attention has not focused sufficiently on other newly emergent infectious diseases which have mortality rates higher than SARS and pandemic influenza.

While the world's attention has been focussed on human cases of bird flu, a far more virulent and dangerous disease was raging through Angola and the Congo, virtually ignored by the rest of the world. An outbreak of Marburg fever, a virulent haemorrhagic fever that was first detected in the late 1960s, broke out in Angola in October 2004 in the remote Uige province in the north of the country. It was only in March 2005 that the Angolan health authorities and the World Health Organization identified the disease for what it was. Marburg is a particularly horrible disease, caused by the same family of viruses that cause Ebola, and there is neither vaccine nor treatment for it. The disease infected 252 people, killing 227 of them before it was finally brought under control a little over a year later. The number of people who were infected and died from this one outbreak of Marburg was greater than those infected by H5N1 influenza. Yet in terms of global attention, the Marburg outbreak was virtually ignored.

Given that its fatality rate was far higher than avian influenza, it could be argued that Marburg was a greater threat to public health and should receive some of the attention and resources that avian influenza is getting. But all diseases are not equal in the global pecking order, and neither are all victims of disease equal. Marburg disease afflicted some of the poorest and weakest people on earth, in a part of the world that is relatively isolated. Marburg disease, though horrible for the victims and their families, is not a major threat to global society. It is not easily transmissible, and there is little likelihood that it will travel to other parts of the world. It has erupted in a remote part of the world, far distanced from the power centres of the global economy.

SARS received the attention it did because unlike most infectious diseases, it affected some of the most highly globalized cities and regions in the world: China, Hong Kong, Singapore, Taiwan, and Toronto. A crisis in these cities and regions is bound to have either a regional or a global impact. Pandemic influenza likewise has assumed the importance it has because the wealthiest and most powerful nations of the world are as vulnerable to the disease as the world's poorest. Migratory birds carrying the H5N1 virus travel across the world, spanning both rich and poor nations. Poultry farms exist everywhere. The combination of migratory birds carrying H5N1 and poultry farms makes it possible for chicken to be infected anywhere, and once chicken are infected, their owners become vulnerable as well. Theoretically, an influenza pandemic can start almost anywhere in the world. And once a pandemic is established anywhere, there is no way to stop it from spreading to other parts except perhaps through a total ban on all local, national, and international travel, a remedy that would probably be more drastic than the disease itself.

There is a danger to ignoring diseases in the remoter parts of the world that do not seem to have any immediate global impact. Besides the moral argument that suffering and disease anywhere in our globalized world requires attention wherever it might occur, self-interest too should indicate that diseases anywhere are a potential threat to people all over the world. The HIV/AIDS virus is most likely to have first passed from animals to humans in the remote rainforests of central Africa, perhaps as early as in the 1930s. For decades, it was a bit like the Marburg virus in Angola: a largely unknown disease in a remote corner of the world. But as far as disease is concerned, in the modern world there are no remote corners. Within a span of decades HIV/AIDS had become the world's leading cause of death from infectious disease.

This is the underlying message that SARS brought to the world: disease is global, and can only be fought on a global level.

Thomas Abraham

ACKNOWLEDGEMENTS

THE seed from which this book grew was planted on a Saturday morning in early May 2003 in the office of Paul K H Tam, Professor of Paediatric Surgery and currently a Pro-Vice-Chancellor of the University of Hong Kong. It was at the height of the SARS epidemic, and like everyone else in Hong Kong, Colin Day, the Publisher of Hong Kong University Press, and I had surgical masks on as we listened to Paul Tam argue the need for a book that would reflect the extraordinary times that the medical profession in Hong Kong was living through. Would not a book aimed at a general audience describing the challenges the medical profession had faced, and explaining the scientific effort that had led to the rapid identification of the SARS coronavirus, be a valuable contribution to public understanding of disease, he asked. It was from that early discussion that this book emerged, though its eventual form has grown from the original concept. Both Paul Tam's original suggestion, as well as Colin Day's continuous support in nurturing this project and helping it grow from idea to book, are gratefully acknowledged. I am also thankful to the Faculty of Medicine at the University of Hong Kong for a grant that made the travel involved in researching this book possible.

This book could not have been written without the generosity of several key players in the SARS story. Malik Peiris, Professor of Virology at the University of Hong Kong, spent long hours explaining the intricacies of life in the viral world and the details of how his team isolated the SARS virus. K Y Yuen, head of the Microbiology Department at the University of Hong Kong, and one of the first doctors in Hong Kong to see a SARS case, shared his experiences and opened doors to other figures, as did K H Chan and John Nicholls. Guan Yi shared his ideas about the origins of the SARS virus. Joseph Sung and Henry Chan at the Prince of Wales Hospital, Andrew Yip at Kwong Wah Hospital, Seto Wing Hong at Queen Mary Hospital, Thomas Tsang at the Department of Health and Osmond Kwok, private practitioner, provided valuable interviews.

David Heymann, then Executive Director of the World Health Organization, helped to organize interviews with the key members of the WHO SARS team, and shared his own experiences. Mike Ryan, head of the WHO's global alert and response network, and Dick Thompson of the WHO press office, provided insights into the international response to SARS, as did Mark Salter, Katrin Leitmeyer and Angela Merianos. Conversations with Henk Bekedam and Alan Schnur of the WHO Beijing office, and Hitoshi Oshitani of the WHO regional office in Manila, during the WHO conference on SARS in Kuala Lumpur in June 2003 provided valuable understanding of the WHO's response to SARS in China.

Meetings with journalists in Guangzhou, who do not wish to be named, provided valuable insights into the way SARS was reported in the media. Qian Gang, a former newspaper editor in Guangzhou and currently Fellow at the Journalism and Media Studies Centre at the University of Hong Kong generously shared his knowledge of the mainland media and some of his research material. Li Cho and Olga Wong, M.Phil candidates at the Journalism and Media Studies Centre, helped with contacts and visits to Guangzhou. Vincent Chen in Guangzhou, and Kelly Chan, an undergraduate at the University of Hong Kong, translated Chinese material.

I owe a debt of gratitude to Yuen Ying Chan, Director of the Journalism and Media Studies Centre, who with characteristic generosity offered me work space, research facilities and encouragement.

My wife, Rebecca, kept our home running and critically read the manuscript unearthing errors and inconsistencies. Our children, Tara and Isaac, patiently put up with their father working seven days a week for the seven months it took to write this book. Without their support this book could not have been written.

1

INTRODUCTION

THE Sunway Lagoon Resort Hotel, half an hour's drive from Kuala Lumpur's international airport, is a large rose stone and glass complex decorated with arches and pillars and surmounted by a minaret-topped dome. The hotel's promotional literature describes it as Malaysia's most versatile convention and exhibition venue, the place to make the ultimate corporate statement. As an added enticement for the jaded convention goer, it also claims the world's largest surf wave pool, a theme park and a huge shopping complex. Despite these multiple attractions, business had been slow in the first half of 2003. The war in Iraq and then the ravages of a new disease, SARS, had kept both the tourists and the convention crowd away. Clearly, no one felt this was quite the right time to make the ultimate corporate statement.

But on June 17 the hotel was buzzing. The carpeted hallways and cavernous conference chambers were crowded with war veterans. They were veterans of wars that few people have heard of. Their battlefields were in places that never made the newspaper headlines: obscure villages and towns with names like Yambuku, Kikwit, Rustaq and Kohlu. And the enemies they fought were too small to see with the naked eye: micro-organisms like the Ebola or the influenza virus. Today though, they were meeting under the full glare of the world's media at a conference organized by the World Health Organization (WHO). A hundred days earlier SARS had swept across the world and suddenly the battles these veterans had fought against microbial disease had become of overwhelming importance to the world, upstaging the more conventional war in Iraq.

The war in Iraq and the invasion of human society by the SARS virus happened at around the same time. The disease first emerged in small outbreaks in southern China in the last few months of 2002, as US and British forces were being deployed in the Persian Gulf in preparation for an invasion. In the second week of March 2003, shortly before the invasion of Iraq on March 20, the SARS virus erupted out of China into the wider world. And as US and British forces ploughed into Iraq, the SARS virus leaped across continents, setting off trails of infection in some of the busiest and most dynamic cities in the world. By some measures, the effects of this new disease were as devastating as a conventional war. By June 2003, over 8000 people had been infected in 32 countries all over the world, and over 900 had died, many of them young and healthy individuals who would normally have expected to live a full life.

The juxtaposition of these two forms of warfare awakened governments to the fact that microbial disease is as great a threat to national security as an invasion by a foreign army. In the US, the anthrax attacks in late 2001 had focused public attention on the way in which disease-causing pathogens could be used as terrorist weapons. But SARS hammered home the message that an infectious disease, even if not intentionally used as a weapon, could be as disruptive and costly as a conventional war. And unlike a conventional war, there was no prior warning of a microbial war: it erupted without notice, and swept though societies that were unprepared to fight it. The head of Hong Kong's public hospital network, Dr William Ho, described SARS as "the Pearl Harbour attack magnified many fold and in a rapidly escalating pattern. We hardly knew anything about the enemy in the beginning."[1]

The analogy of war echoed throughout the SARS crisis. This was an attack by an unseen invader to which nations had to respond as they would to any other attack — by mobilizing the resources to repel the invader. For many countries it became clear that the real threat to security would come not from invading armies, but from unknown microbes. "We must remember that in this region, we are more likely to be invaded by microbes than by a foreign army," Malaysia's Health Minister Chua Jui Meng pointed out.[2]

This war by microbes targeted the vital infrastructure of society; in this case, the public health system. The virus first hit doctors, nurses and health care workers, mowing them down like soldiers on a battlefield. But unlike soldiers who are trained to face death, medical workers are trained to save lives. Without warning they found themselves thrown onto the front lines of a battle in which they were the cannon fodder. And like a guerrilla fighter, the SARS virus managed to turn public health systems to its own advantage: spreading in hospitals and finding new victims who would in turn take the disease out into the wider community. Not only was this a disease for which modern medicine had no cure, it was a disease that used the institutions of modern medicine to spread.

In the areas hit hardest by SARS, people experienced a fear their forefathers had lived with constantly: the dread of death from disease. The ghosts of an era when death from epidemics of plague, pneumonia and influenza was as routine as the changing of the seasons had returned to haunt a generation that had grown to believe that modern medicine had vanquished infectious diseases.

The economic cost of the disease was also devastating. In a little over three months, SARS touched every continent, and paralyzed some of the world's most dynamic cities and regions. The global economy lost about US$30 billion in production, most of it in Asia. Governments clamped quarantines and other restrictions on travellers, reversing a decades-long global trend of loosening travel restrictions. Airports emptied, airlines cancelled flights and it appeared as if the virus had blocked the arteries of a networked, interconnected, globalized twenty-first century world.

Gro Harlem Brundtland, the then Director-General of the WHO, summed up the impact that a minute virus could have on the world:

> We are dealing with a new disease striking a globalized society. We have seen its rapid international spread. We have seen stock markets move up or down according to the latest success or setback in the SARS situation. We have seen bustling transportation hubs go silent. We have seen SARS on the front pages and on our TV screens. We have seen the closure of hospitals, schools and borders. We have seen economic impact, population movements from affected cities and unwarranted discrimination.[3]

By June, when health experts from all over the world met in Malaysia, the worst of the epidemic was over. In three of the initial outbreak centres, Hong Kong, Vietnam and Singapore, there had been no recent cases of the disease. In Toronto, another of the cities to be hit hard by SARS, the outbreak was coming under control. It was only in mainland China and Taiwan that new cases were still being reported. But here too, the number of new cases was falling, and it was apparent that the epidemic was dying out. There was an understandable air of self-congratulation and mutual back-patting among the scientists and public health officials. Clearly, much had been achieved in 100 days. The epidemic had slowed, the virus causing the disease had been identified, a great deal had been learned about its method of transmission and significant clinical knowledge had been gathered on how best to treat the disease.

But there were also many disturbing, unanswered questions. How was it possible that at the beginning of the twenty-firt century, with the armamentarium of modern medicine at its disposal, humankind was still so vulnerable to disease-causing microbes? If this disease had erupted without warning and ambushed the world with such devastating effects, were there other new diseases waiting to attack in a similar way? Were we facing a century of new diseases?

* * *

Joshua Lederberg is a towering figure in the world of contemporary microbiology. He won the Nobel Prize in 1958 at the age of 33 for his work on genetic recombination in bacteria. For several decades, he has been a leading, and often lonely, voice warning of the threat to human society posed by viruses. "The threat of a major virus epidemic — a global pandemic, hangs over the head of the species at any time," he wrote in 1968.[4] This was after a previously unknown virus infected 37 people in Marburg and Frankfurt in Germany, and in Belgrade, Yugoslavia, killing five of them. The virus had been transmitted to humans by African green monkeys being transported from Uganda to laboratories in Germany. The symptoms of the disease were horrifying. Patients' skin, hair and nails peeled off, blood erupted from every orifice and within two weeks the constant internal and external bleeding led to multiple organ failure.[5]

Because the disease broke out in a laboratory environment, it was contained before it had a chance to spread to the larger community. But for Lederberg, this was a classic example of the danger that the viral world posed to human society. A pandemic caused by exotic lethal viruses from the animal kingdom was an event for which the world needed to be prepared. And if the virus was virulent and readily transmissible, a worst-case scenario would be the decimation of the human race. "The survival of the human population is not a preordained evolutionary programme," he warned. The human presence on earth was challenged only by microbes, "the predator for which we remain the prey."[6]

In the case of the Marburg virus, Lederberg felt the world had a near miss. Rather than infecting human beings in a laboratory in Germany, the virus could "easily have established a large focus of infection in countries like India or China or South Vietnam, and in our present knowledge of virology, we would have been ill equipped to stop it from dominating the earth, with a half a billion casualties."[7]

In the late 1960s, Lederberg's apocalyptic warnings went against the contemporary belief that infectious diseases no longer posed a threat to humankind. The discovery of penicillin by Alexander Fleming in 1928 and its mass production in the post-war years seemed to mark a decisive turning point in the human battle against infectious diseases. Penicillin and other antibiotics proved to be miraculously effective against an array of previously lethal bacterial diseases, including the plague, tuberculosis and pneumonia. Mortality rates from infectious diseases fell rapidly in the developed world and life expectancies rose. While viral diseases were resistant to antibiotics, antiviral drugs that targeted essential proteins required by viruses to cause infection soon arrived on the market. While the antivirals were not always effective, it only seemed a matter of time before science would make it possible to treat viral diseases with drugs in the way that bacterial diseases were treated.

Using these new drugs as well as vaccination, plans were laid in the 1950s and 60s to eradicate malaria, polio, tuberculosis and smallpox globally. The WHO declared that these diseases, which had afflicted humans from the earliest times, would soon be eradicated. Infectious diseases appeared to be a thing of the past, and the US Surgeon General reflected the spirit of the age when he declared in 1969 that "we can now close the book on infectious disease."[8]

The decades that followed proved him to be spectacularly wrong. As the twentieth century came to a close, it became apparent that with the exception of smallpox, which had been eliminated through a global vaccination campaign, all of the diseases targeted for eradication 40 years earlier were still flourishing. Tuberculosis remained one of the three largest causes of infectious disease deaths in the world, killing an estimated 1.6 million people a year. Roughly 2 billion people, or nearly a third of the world's population, were thought to be carrying the tuberculosis bacillus, though the majority would not develop the disease. Malaria was also resurgent, particularly in Africa.[9]

It was not merely that efforts to eradicate these diseases had failed. The organisms that caused these diseases had returned in new, drug-resistant forms. Penicillin, the first of the post-war wonder drugs, was also the first to become ineffective in the face of new generations of penicillin-resistant bacteria. Then other antibiotics began to fail as well. Soon experts began to predict the imminent arrival of a post-antibiotic age, when all the common antibiotics would cease to be effective.[10]

Besides the return of old diseases in new, drug-resistant forms, the last few decades of the twentieth century also saw the emergence of a host of new viral diseases, of which HIV/AIDS is the best-known. In the 20 years since the disease was identified, it has spread across the globe and become the largest public health threat now facing the world.

By 2003, there were an estimated 40 million people worldwide infected with the HIV virus, which was continuing to spread at a devastating rate. The WHO estimated that 14 000 people a day were contracting AIDS. But HIV/AIDS is only one of nearly 20 new diseases that have emerged since the 1970s. Of these, Ebola is the most lethal, with a fatality rate of over 80 percent. Others, like Nipah, Hendra and Hantavirus pulmonary syndrome, produce lower mortality rates, but like Ebola, have no cure. Lederberg's warnings about the threat posed by new viral diseases suddenly appeared remarkably prescient. During the 1980s and 90s, the study of emerging infectious diseases became the focus of urgent attention in the US, leading to a series of scientific reports warning of the threat posed by new microbes, and suggesting appropriate protective measures.[11]

Lederberg and other scientists saw viruses as being uniquely dangerous for a number of reasons. First, unlike bacteria, against which newer generations of antibiotics could be developed, the very nature of a virus makes it far more difficult to develop effective antiviral drugs. Viral evolutionary patterns also result in the faster generation of mutant varieties than is the case with bacteria, making viruses a rapidly shifting target for both the human immune system and the manufacturers of vaccines and antiviral drugs.

Viruses evoke the same kinds of emotions in us as the great white shark or the giant carnivores from the age of the dinosaurs: a mixture of awe and terror at a form of life that is so basic, yet so perfectly suited to its ultimate purpose of preying on other forms of life. Unlike bacteria, which are large enough to possess all the biological mechanisms needed for independent life, viruses are the ultimate parasites. They are little more than minute ribbons of DNA or RNA wrapped in a protein casing. Viruses have no metabolism and they lack the ability to reproduce independently. As the microbiologist Dorothy Crawford put it, "viruses represent life stripped to the bare essentials."[12]

A virus comes to life only after it enters a living cell, whether a plant cell, an animal cell or even a bacteria. Once the virus penetrates the host cell, it engineers a molecular coup d'etat, and takes over the cell's machinery, which it then uses to reproduce itself. In the process, the host cell is severely weakened and eventually dies. The virus however, has achieved its purpose by using the cell to create thousands of copies of itself. It is the fundamental incompatibility of the aim of the virus, which is to find a host and take over its cells to manufacture new viruses, and the aim of the host, which is to preserve its own life, that makes the relationship between host and virus a battle, manifested as disease.

But the interaction between host and virus does not always lead to disease. Long-term adversaries often come to an agreement to live and let live, and this is what tends to happen over the long-run between a virus and its host. Most living creatures carry viral parasites with which they have lived and evolved over the centuries to reach a state of accommodation. The virus lives and reproduces within its natural host without causing the host any apparent harm. Most evolutionary biologists believe that this kind of symbiotic relationship is the equilibrium towards which virus and host evolve. It is not in the virus' interest to weaken the host so much that it dies prematurely: this forces the virus to find a constant supply of new hosts, and if that is not possible, the virus itself will die out. As Lederberg observed, "the host rapidly destroyed is a pyrrhic victory for the parasite."[13] A better relationship is one in which the virus can reproduce over a long period of time within a healthy host.

The process of accommodation between virus and host can take centuries of co evolution. Severe viral diseases tend to occur when viruses meet new hosts for the first time. Virus and host are unfamiliar with each other, and the reaction is strong. The host usually has no immunity to the new virus, often leading to fatal disease. All of the new viral diseases that have cropped up over the last few decades have been zoonotic, meaning they are caused when viruses that normally live in animal hosts jump to human hosts, causing severe infection.

The reasons for the increase in these kinds of encounters during the past 30 years lie in the disturbances to previously untouched ecosystems caused by human activity.[14] Building roads and clearing virgin forests, for example, brings humans in contact with new viral species living in animals and insects. If a virus can jump from its host species to a human host, the result will be a viral infection. As we multiply and expand across the planet, occupying new areas of the earth's surface, the chances of encountering new infectious agents continues to increase. And we have been multiplying and expanding at a staggering rate, particularly over the last 100 years. In 1900, the earth's human population stood at around 1.6 billion. By 2000, there were over 6.3 billion people. By 2050, the earth will have to support an estimated 9 billion people.

These exploding numbers have led humans to enter ecosystems they have never entered before: jungles and forests have been cleared, swamps drained, roads constructed and towns and cities built in environments where animals, plants and microbes had lived stable, settled existences isolated from human advances for thousands of years. In the same way that a wasps' nest is disturbed by a carelessly poked stick, human intrusion disturbs a variety of delicately balanced ecological relationships. And just as a swarm of angry wasps will attack an intruder, viruses, bacteria, parasites and insects respond to human intrusion by attempting to jump from their natural host to man. More often than not, they do not succeed. But when they do, the result can be a new infectious disease.

It usually takes more than a virus jumping from an animal to a human host to create an epidemic. The virus must be able to move easily between humans, and not merely occasionally from animals to humans. Fortunately, most of the new disease-causing viruses that have emerged in recent decades have been animal viruses that have not quite perfected their strategy for hopping from human to human. So while they may cause fearsome disease among those they infect, the disease rarely spreads far. The exceptions have been AIDS and SARS, both diseases caused by a virus with the ability to transmit easily between humans.

But even more than the nature of the virus, it is our own cultural and social practices — the way we live, the food we eat, our relationship with the environment — that create the conditions for a new disease-causing virus to gain a foothold and spread in the human population.

Consider the case of HIV/AIDS, which erupted almost simultaneously in the US and Africa in the early 1980s, and then raged across the world, mowing down young, healthy men and women to become the world's leading cause of death from infectious disease. The origins of HIV/AIDS are still shrouded in controversy, but the general consensus is that the HIV virus first passed to humans from monkeys in the rainforests of Central Africa.[15]

The HIV virus is related to a group of viruses known as the simian immunodeficiency viruses (SIV), which are found among a variety of monkeys and chimpanzees in the equatorial forests of Africa. The closest relative to HIV1, which causes the most virulent form of AIDS in humans, is a SIV virus that has been found in a few chimpanzees in Gabon and Zaire in the same area where the first human HIV cases were recorded.

Researchers who have tried to reconstruct the evolution of the virus have suggested that HIV could have first appeared in humans as early as the 1930s, when it was passed from captured chimpanzees to hunters through bites and cuts. Following these initial encounters, the virus continued to evolve over the decades, adapting to the human body, becoming more adept at transmitting between humans. At the same time, contact between hunters and chimpanzees increased as roads built by logging companies opened up the rainforest and the demand for "bush meat" increased in the towns and cities of West and Central Africa.

The virus probably caused isolated epidemics among humans in small, rural African communities. But it had already begun to travel. In 1976, a Norwegian sailor who had travelled to West Africa died of a mysterious disease. His wife, who contracted the same disease, died as well. Years later, after AIDS had been identified as a new disease, their tissue samples were tested and found to be HIV-positive. Going further back in time, blood samples from a 48-year-old sailor who had died in New York in 1959 showed signs of HIV infection, as did samples from a 15-year-old boy who had died in St Louis, Missouri, in 1968. These isolated cases of the disease never exploded into an epidemic. It required major shifts in human behaviour to create the conditions for the virus to transmit between humans at a rate high enough to cause an epidemic.

The HIV virus is transmitted through bodily fluids, primarily blood and semen. In the US, the 1970s saw a fundamental shift in social mores that would provide the virus with an environment in which it could explode into an epidemic. This was a period when sexual behaviour in general was liberated from earlier constraints. And no one embraced this liberation more than the male homosexual community, which came out en masse in a series of gay pride marches and celebrated its new-found sexual confidence in an orgy of activity in bathhouses and clubs in New York and San Francisco, the two capitals of the gay liberation movement.

Anonymous sex with multiple partners as often as possible became a fundamental element of gay liberation. This provided an ideal environment for sexually transmitted diseases in general, and the HIV virus in particular, to transmit rapidly from human to human.

A second critical factor in the HIV/AIDS epidemic was the sharp explosion in the number of heroin users and the sharing of unsterilized needles, creating another environment in which a virus transmitted through blood could multiply rapidly. Overlap between the drug using and the male homosexual community allowed the virus to multiply in both groups.

A third source of new hosts for the virus was blood banks, which purchased blood from professional donors who were more often than not down and out drug addicts who needed money for their next fix. Until the late 1980s, when screening and treatment of blood and plasma supplies became routine, the virus was passed on from infected donors to blood recipients. These three elements: sexual liberation, increased drug use and sharing of needles and blood donations provided the social and cultural backdrop for the AIDS epidemic in the US.

In Africa, the conditions that gave rise to the epidemic were different. Here, it was the armed conflicts, wars and economic upheavals of post-colonial Africa that created the social conditions for the virus to spread. During the 1970s and 80s, the Great Lakes region of Central Africa, which includes Zaire, Uganda, Tanzania, Rwanda and Burundi, was one of the most unstable areas in the world. The movement of soldiers, particularly between Tanzania and Uganda, and the disruption of traditional economies that sent men to search for work in urban centres, and women into prostitution in towns along major road and river routes, encouraged promiscuity and created the conditions for a virus that had previously affected only isolated communities to spread across Sub-Saharan Africa.

Besides transmitting sexually, the virus also spread in Africa due to poorly equipped hospitals and the repeated re-use of needles in much the same way that it had spread as a result of the sharing of needles among drug addicts in the West. Throughout history, social disruptions and economic distress have provided fertile soil for diseases to flourish. The spread of AIDS in Africa is only the latest example of this phenomenon.

The origins and epidemiology of HIV/AIDS are particularly complex and politically sensitive. In the case of other emerging diseases, the link between human intervention in natural ecosystems and the emergence of disease is more straightforward, as the story of the Nipah virus illustrates.[16] In 1997, giant forest fires broke out in Kalimantan and Borneo in Indonesia, blanketing the region in acrid clouds of smoke. Large-scale burning of the forests to clear land for plantations and agriculture had sparked the fires, which spread rapidly due to unusually dry conditions caused by the El Nino effect. By the time the fires had burned out, 9.7 million hectares of forest land had been charred and 75 million people had been affected in some way or another.

But the fires were to have long-term consequences as well. In the autumn of 1998, a mysterious illness broke out in the Malaysian state of Perak. The early symptoms, high fever and muscle pains, were similar to flu. As the disease progressed however, the brain tissues of patients became inflamed, leading to convulsions and eventually coma. Doctors first thought the disease was Japanese encephalitis. But vaccination against encephalitis did little to stop its spread. No drugs seemed to work, and almost half of those who developed symptoms died.

One interesting feature of the outbreak offered a clue as to its cause:

many of those who had fallen ill worked on pig farms, and pigs on these farms were also falling ill and dying. Analysis of samples from pigs and humans revealed that a previously unknown virus from the paramyxovirus family, the same family of viruses that causes measles, was responsible. The natural host of the virus was found to be the Malaysian flying fox, *Pteropus vammpyrus,* a giant bat with a five-foot wing span that normally lives deep in the jungles of Southeast Asia, far from human civilization. However, these bats had been noticed eating mango fruit from the trees around the pig farms where the disease had broken out. After feasting on the fruit, the bats had dropped half-eaten mangos covered with their virus-laden saliva on to the ground. The pigs in turn had eaten the fruit and contracted the virus, which they had then passed on to workers on the farms.

What had prompted these normally forest-dwelling flying foxes to come so close to human habitation to feed? Researchers believe the most likely explanation is that the bats' unusual behaviour was triggered by smog from the forest fires the previous year. The smoke and the fire had prevented the fruit trees in the bat's normal habitat from flowering, so the bats had flown nearly a thousand kilometres to find food in the fruit trees of Perak.[17] Like the apocryphal flap of the butterfly's wing in China that triggered a storm in New York, an event in the forests of Indonesia had led to the emergence of a new disease in Malaysia.

Human behaviour has led to the emergence of new diseases. Human technology, in the form of global air travel, has made it possible for these diseases to spread around the world faster than ever before. The greatest boon for viruses, bacteria and other micro-organisms seeking new hosts has been the rapid growth of air travel. As SARS demonstrated, the speed of modern air travel ensures that a virus that is in Hong Kong today can be carried by a sick traveller to any point in Southeast Asia within 3 or 4 hours, to Europe in 12 hours and to North America in 18 hours. Nearly 1.5 billion passengers travel by air every year, creating countless opportunities for diseases to spread rapidly across the globe.

Contrast this with the rate at which disease travelled in earlier centuries. In 1827, the second cholera pandemic of the nineteenth century broke out in India. It was carried to Afghanistan and the borders of Russia in 1827 by traders, and arrived in Moscow in 1830. Merchants then carried the disease to other European cities by 1831. Thanks to the recently introduced steamboat service across the Atlantic, the cholera bacteria reached North America in 1832 and spread through Canada and the US.[18] The disease took five years to travel from India to North America. Given this time frame, outbreaks in one part of the world had died down before the disease appeared in other parts of the world. If an epidemic of an equally virulent disease broke out today, it could cross the globe in less than a day, and every continent would be battling it simultaneously.

It is not only humans who transport disease-carrying organisms to new locations. Animals and plants do so as well, as a recent example from the US shows. In the 1990s, American pet owners who wanted something more exotic than the cat, dog or hamster owned by their neighbours but were not prepared to go as far as keeping a boa constrictor or an alligator found a happy alternative in the Gambian giant rat. These large rodents, native to large parts of Sub-Saharan Africa, were attractive enough in appearance (one website devoted to the creature gushed, "they have an absolutely adorable face, actually rather comical and whimsical in appearance. If you like rodents, they are sure to captivate you in a heartbeat"[19]) and sufficiently docile to become desirable novelty pets in the US.

In its natural environment, the Gambian giant rat, like every other living creature, is host to a variety of bacteria, viruses and other parasites that it has evolved with over generations and which cause it no harm. When the rats were transported over oceans and across continents, these microbes went with them.

In April 2003, a consignment of Gambian giant rats destined for pet shops in the US was shipped from Ghana to a dealer in Texas.[20] One of the rats was sold to a pet dealer in the Mid-West, who housed it together with a collection of prairie dogs, large rodents that normally live on the Great Plains of the US but have now been domesticated as pets.

On May 11, a 28-year-old Wisconsin woman, Tammy Kautzer, bought two of the prairie dogs for her three-year-old daughter Schyan.[21] Two days later, one of the creatures fell sick, and its eyes began oozing fluid and later crusted over. The out-of-sorts animal also bit the little girl on her right index finger. The prairie dog became sicker and eventually died; the little girl developed a high fever and pox-like blisters formed on her head, hands and feet. Soon, her parents developed the same symptoms.

Public health authorities, who had been on the alert for possible terrorist attacks using biological weapons ever since the September 11 attacks, were alarmed by the fact that three people were showing symptoms that bore an eerie resemblance to smallpox, one of the diseases it was feared that potential terrorists could use.

Blood and tissue samples from the three patients were sent to the Centre for Diseases Control and Prevention (CDC) in Atlanta for analysis. The results contained good news as well as bad. The good news was that the disease was not smallpox. The worrying news was that these were the first reported cases outside Africa of monkeypox, a disease caused by a virus from the smallpox family. Monkeypox cases normally occur in isolated communities in the Central and West African rainforests. The virus lives in rainforest primates and squirrels and is passed on to humans through cuts and bites.

Working backwards, researchers found that one of the Gambian giant rats had infected the prairie dogs with the monkeypox virus, which had then passed it on to the human patients.[22] Monkeypox is generally a mild disease, and Schyan and her parents survived little worse for their experience. But by the end of July 2003, there were over 70 suspected human cases in the US, all transmitted through contact with prairie dogs that had been infected by Gambian giant rats.

In today's globalized world it is increasingly easy for a virus to be transported out of its natural environment to new areas where it can spread and find new hosts to infect. The monkeypox virus from the rainforests of Central Africa has now found a potential new host among the large prairie dog population in the US. If the monkeypox virus and prairie dogs adapt to each other, the disease could become endemic in the US.

At least one exotic disease has already become endemic in the US in recent years, West Nile virus fever. In 1999, the first case of the fever, which is found in Uganda and Egypt, was reported in New York. By 2002, the virus, which is present in birds and other animals and transmitted to humans by mosquitoes, had spread to 44 states in the US, infecting 4000 people and killing 284.[23]

These kinds of encounters between humans and viruses have been going on throughout human history.[24] At every stage of human evolution, new viruses have passed from animals to man. When hunter-gatherers learned to domesticate animals and began to settle in agricultural communities, viruses from cattle passed to humans, causing diseases like measles and smallpox. Later, as urban civilizations developed, the presence of tens of thousands of people living in close proximity to one another in towns and cities gave viruses the opportunity to infect large numbers of people rapidly in the form of epidemics. Now, our globalized world has made the spread of disease on a pandemic scale easier than ever before.

But if this process has been going on throughout human history, what is there to be worried about? The emergence of a new virus in the human population is, for the reasons we saw earlier, marked by a particularly fierce battle between human host and virus, leading to huge loss of life. Over time, virus and host reach an accommodation, and the disease symptoms become progressively milder, or even disappear. Today, measles is a mild childhood disease. But when it first emerged in the human population, it was terrifyingly lethal. Over the centuries, it has become progressively milder as virus and host have co-evolved.

New viral diseases have emerged throughout history, and their emergence has often been accompanied by lethal epidemics. A new virus emerging today could cause the same kind of devastation that smallpox and measles caused in the Roman Empire and in other early civilizations. While the means at our disposal to fight disease are infinitely more sophisticated than they have ever been in human history, we are still uniquely vulnerable to viral diseases, as HIV/AIDS and Ebola have shown.

SARS was a warning to the world of what a new virus could do. Because it was transmitted easily from person to person, it was also able to take advantage of the speed of modern air travel and spread rapidly across the globe. The good news was that even though it spread relatively easily through droplets from infected persons, it did not spread as easily as some other diseases, such as influenza. The influenza virus can travel a relatively long distance through the air, and the average influenza sufferer infects at least 10 people. Droplet-borne SARS viruses, on the other hand, rarely travel more than several metres, restricting its transmission, with a few notable exceptions, to people who have been in close contact with a SARS patient.

SARS had a fatality rate of around 11 percent, high by the standards of most common diseases. The case fatality rate for normal strains of influenza, for example, is around 1 percent, and this is mostly among the elderly and infirm. But SARS was not as lethal as Ebola, which has a mortality rate of between 70 and 90 percent. The nightmare for the human race would be a new disease with the transmissibility of influenza and the lethality of Ebola. This would be a disease with the potential to spread widely and kill the majority of those who contracted it. This is the kind of pandemic that Lederberg and others have been warning of as a threat to human society.

The world was lucky with SARS. It was fairly lethal, but not uncontrollably so. It was fairly transmissible, but once again not uncontrollably so. Given the rate at which new infectious diseases have been cropping up, the probability that a virus that is more lethal and more transmissible than SARS will emerge is increasing. The chapters that follow look at how SARS emerged, how it spread, how it was fought and its impact on the societies it hit the hardest. In understanding these issues, we are also gaining lessons on how to prevent a more lethal pandemic in the future.

2

CHINA

FEBRUARY 1, 2003 was the first day of Chinese New Year, according to the Chinese calendar, the beginning of the Year of the Goat. It was a day on which Fan Xinde, a 57-year-old ambulance driver in the southern Chinese city of Guangzhou, would normally not have been at work. The New Year period is traditionally a time for family reunions, and Fan should have been with his wife, Yu Meiji, a hospital nutritionist, and their 27-year-old son, Fan Weibin. But as chance would have it, one of his fellow ambulance drivers at the Second Affiliated Hospital of Zhongshan University in Guangzhou had recently lost his mother and wanted to spend New Year's Day with his bereaved father. So Fan agreed to fill in for him.[1]

At about 10.15 a.m. Fan was told to transfer a critically ill patient to the Third Affiliated Hospital a few kilometres away. He was warned that the patient was extremely infectious and given a triple-layer surgical mask and gloves to wear. Masked and gloved, he loaded the sick man into the back of the ambulance and helped to adjust his oxygen flow. During the short journey, the patient struggled for breath, vomiting and spewing phlegm and mucous in the ambulance. When Fan got back to the Second Affiliated Hospital, he spent an hour or so scrubbing the ambulance and disinfecting it.

Three days later, on February 4, Fan began to feel feverish while at work. He was kept in the hospital for observation, and phoned his wife to let her know. She was puzzled at his falling ill, but not unduly alarmed. When she got to the hospital with food and clothes for him, she found Fan feverish but otherwise well. But when she returned to see him the next day, she was shocked. Fan, a large man, was so weak that he could not walk to the toilet unaided. He needed help even drinking a glass of water.

The ambulance driver's condition deteriorated, and X-rays showed patches on his lungs that were growing at an alarming rate. The doctors treated him with antibiotics, but his lungs became increasingly inflamed and filled with fluid. His fever would not come down, and nothing the doctors did seemed to help. On February 10, six days after being admitted to hospital, Fan was unable to breathe on his own and was transferred to the Intensive Care Unit (ICU), where he was put on a mechanical ventilator. Day by day the disease continued to destroy the delicate tissue of his lungs, starving his body of oxygen. After battling to stay alive for 20 days, Fan Xinde, a man described by those who knew him as "an ordinary man, a simple Guangdong person," died on February 24, his body unable to survive the destruction of his lungs. History would record him as the first medical worker to die of SARS in an epidemic that eventually infected over 1700 health care workers worldwide.[2]

His 60-year-old wife, who had been caring for him in hospital, also fell ill with SARS. She had been looking after her husband in hospital, feeding and nursing him until he was taken to the ICU. No one had warned her about how infectious the disease was, so she did not wear a mask or any protective clothing. This was a pattern that would be repeated in the next few months in different parts of the world. Because they knew nothing about the disease, those who contracted it would unwittingly pass it onto their relatives and friends, with often tragic results. Fortunately, Yu Meiji's illness was less severe than her husband's, and she survived.

As Fan lay critically ill, panic was spreading through the Second Affiliated Hospital. The day he was admitted, other hospital workers were falling sick with the same symptoms. At first, doctors and nurses on the 12th floor respiratory illness ward fell ill. Then patients on the ward caught the disease. Next, it travelled to the 13th and 15th floors. The disease spread relentlessly; within two weeks, 93 hospital staff, patients and relatives had fallen ill.[3]

Hospitals deal with disease constantly, and doctors and nurses occasionally fall ill. But they rarely fall ill at the same time and in such large numbers. Most illnesses that require hospitalization are not infectious enough to spread easily to hospital staff. And even when they are infectious, standard infection control procedures such as washing hands and wearing gloves and masks prevent the disease from spreading from patient to carer. But in the case of this new disease, even wearing masks did not seem to help.

No one had seen a disease that spread so fast; hit young, healthy people so hard; and was so resistant to antibiotics. And there was no clue as to what was causing it. Analysis of nasal and bronchial swabs as well as blood and serum samples from patients did not reveal any of the known respiratory disease-causing pathogens. Pneumonia is normally the result of an infection by one of many common bacteria: *Streptococcus pneumoniae*, various forms of *Legionella* bacteria, *Mycoplasma pneumoniae* or *Chlamydia pneumoniae*, to name a few. All of these infections are easily treatable by antibiotics. This disease did not respond to antibiotics, and so was probably viral. But tests for the viruses that can cause pneumonia-like symptoms, including the flu virus, proved to be negative.

As hospital epidemiologists searched for the source of the infection, they made an astounding discovery: a single patient had been responsible for setting off this chain of infection. He was the patient that Fan had transferred in his ambulance, Zhou Zuofeng, a 46-year-old seafood trader. Zhou, whom medical staff would dub the "poison king," had only spent around 18 hours at the Second Affiliated Hospital, but in that time he had directly infected 28 hospital staff, who in turn passed the infection on to other colleagues and to patients.

Zhou also set off smaller clusters of infection at the two other hospitals to which he was transferred. At the Third Affiliated Hospital, 23 doctors and nurses and 18 patients and their relatives were infected. At the Eighth Municipal People's Hospital, he infected another 20 health care workers.

The chains of infection that Zhou set off in three of Guangzhou's biggest hospitals in the first week of February sparked alarm among doctors. From what they had seen so far, this disease was a public health nightmare: it was a highly contagious respiratory ailment of unknown cause and with no known treatment, spreading rapidly through the hospital system.

As news of doctors and nurses being infected with a mystery disease trickled out, the public became alarmed. Officially, there was not a word from the hospital authorities or the Guangdong provincial health department about the situation. But word got out as health care workers told their friends and families about the crisis they were facing. The people of Guangzhou also sensed that authorities were worried about a crisis situation. At the height of the New Year holiday season, masked policemen appeared at Guangzhou Railway Station among the holiday travellers, moving people along and trying to prevent crowds from gathering. It was only later that people would realize that this was because there was an outbreak of a contagious disease in the city, and the government was trying to reduce the risk of it spreading in crowded places.

There was no news about the disease in the official media, so the citizens of Guangzhou began sending each other SMS messages sharing whatever information they had. One message that was circulated on February 6 said that 105 people had been infected with the disease, 44 of whom had already died, and that the Third Affiliated Hospital had been closed to the public. Other messages urged people to boil vinegar as the fumes would act as a disinfectant, and to stock up on *banlangen*, a Chinese herbal medicine used to treat colds and fevers. As the messages and the rumours spread, this triggered panic buying of vinegar and *banlangen*. Queues formed outside pharmacies in Guangzhou, and canny shopkeepers responded by raising the prices of their products to meet this sudden demand. Bottles of vinegar that normally sold for a couple of *yuan* were now being sold for 100 *yuan*, and as supplies ran out, one newspaper reported that a bottle had been sold for 1000 *yuan*. Packets of *banlangen* that sold for 10 *yuan* were being sold for three and four times that price. Erythromycin, a common antibiotic, was in great demand, as were surgical masks.

Newspapers and radio and television stations maintained a complete silence as rumours and panic continued to spread. Journalists in Guangzhou were aware that something serious was happening. Many had friends and contacts who were doctors who told them about the panic in the hospitals. The journalists reported the situation to their editors, but this was not a story that could be reported easily. On February 8, two of Guangzhou's major newspapers, the *Nanfang Daily* and the *Yangcheng Wanbao*, carried short news reports about a "mysterious illness" that had hit the hospitals in Guangzhou. The propaganda department of the provincial Communist Party, which oversees the media, acted quickly to prevent further media coverage. The same day it sent the first of a series of notices to media organizations asking them not to cover the disease to avoid "public fear and instability."[4]

The press in Guangdong province is outspoken by Chinese standards. While all media in China is state-controlled, the rapid opening up of the Chinese economy and the push to develop a modern media industry has led to an increase in media autonomy. Though still subject to the overall control of the Communist Party propaganda department, many newspapers are no longer funded by the state, and instead make their money commercially by attracting readers and advertisers. This has encouraged newspaper managers to build readership through increasingly bold reporting and commentary, though usually within the limits of what the authorities consider acceptable. While criticism of senior leaders and questioning of party policy is taboo, media outlets are increasingly able to report on corruption and a variety of other social issues.

Guangdong province, which has a number of media groups vigorously competing for readers, has probably gone the furthest in pushing the boundaries on press freedom. So when the propaganda department sent its first notice on February 8, newspapers continued to send reporters to hospitals to interview doctors and hospital administrators about what was happening. On February 10, the propaganda department sent out a further directive asking news outlets not to send reporters to hospitals or interview doctors and patients about the disease. On February 12, another directive was issued banning reporting on panic buying of food and medicine. The only reports that could be published were official press releases from government departments.

Reporters, however, continued to go to hospitals and talk to doctors and senior hospital administrators, who were happy enough to let others know about the emergency they were facing. But some of the information gathered was not published until media restrictions were eased a few months later. The Nanfang group of newspapers in particular tried to push the boundaries of censorship by finding ways to report indirectly on the situation. This was done by reporting on aspects of the outbreak that the press was not explicitly prohibited from covering. When, for example, early directives banned interviewing doctors, newspapers and media outlets reported on panic buying. When this was also prohibited, they reported on official action taken against traders who were profiting from the scare buying.

Often, these reports were presented as efforts to clear up rumours about the disease. But in reporting official efforts to quell rumours, the media also managed to give the public an idea of the content of these so-called rumours. For example, on February 12, the *Nanfang Daily* published a detailed account of how the epidemic had broken out in various provincial towns in Guangdong before spreading to the capital of Guangzhou. But instead of saying that the disease was spreading, the newspaper reported on how rumours about the disease had spread, in the process giving a detailed account of what the rumours were saying. In order to indicate that the disease had begun to spread in Guangzhou at the beginning of February, the newspaper reported that, "From the beginning of February, the rumour about an epidemic began to spread in Guangzhou." The article went on to describe the symptoms of the disease and mentioned its high infectivity, but again, as if reporting a rumour. "The typical version of the rumour said ... the symptoms of the epidemic included fever and patches on the lungs, and within a day respiratory failure appeared. The rumour also said that the disease was incurable and that many patients died." [5]

In this way, playing a cat and mouse game with the provincial propaganda authorities, the media was able to pass on driblets of information to the public. But by February 19, the authorities had had enough of this and issued a blanket prohibition on reporting on any aspect of the situation except those details provided in official communiqués. On the same day, the propaganda department issued a further directive specifying that nothing about the epidemic could be reported. Reporting on the number of cases and the causes of the disease, interviewing experts and publishing their views and even the use of the term "atypical pneumonia" was prohibited except in official press releases.

In the absence of credible news reports, rumours swirled and panic spread. Besides buying medicines, people also began stocking up on basic food items like rice, salt and oil. Other provinces began to experience a shortage of medicines due to consumer demands in Guangzhou. As far away as Chengdu, the capital of Szechuan province in central China, supplies of *banlangen* and vinegar were running short as supplies were diverted to Guangdong in response to the higher prices there.

Fear soon seeped out into the neighbouring provinces. A rumour that a sick person from Guangzhou had taken the disease to Hainan, an island province about 300 kilometres to the south, sparked a run on vinegar and Chinese medicines in towns throughout the province.

On February 10, an SMS message began circulating in Guangzhou that would trigger alarm internationally. The anonymous message said that the disease was caused by a mutant influenza virus, and that the anti-influenza drug Tamiflu was the best cure. The message caught the attention of the World Health Organization (WHO) global influenza surveillance network. If a mutant flu virus was causing an epidemic, this was a matter of serious global concern, and the WHO wanted to know about it. On February 10, the WHO's regional office in Manila sent a message to the Central government in Beijing, asking for information about the epidemic. This would be the first of many international attempts to obtain information about the disease from Chinese authorities.

Why did the Guangdong provincial government try to hide the disease? There were several reasons. The Chinese political system prizes stability and order above all else, and any news that could spark public panic, or dissatisfaction with the government, is suppressed. Diseases and disasters are both seen by the Communist Party as "negative news." The recent efforts to discourage reporting on the spread of HIV/AIDS in China are typical of the attitude of the Party and the government towards reporting major public health problems. A less well-known cover up occurred in 1988 during a major outbreak of Hepatitis A in Shanghai, during which over 300 000 people were infected, and over 30 died. The hospital system in Shanghai was overwhelmed by the numbers of patients, but the media was not allowed to report this story. Often the cover-up is started by local government officials, who do not want to get in trouble with their higher-ups. "Actually to delay reporting about diseases is almost a tradition in China, partially because of officialism and localism," comments Yin Xiaorong, an assistant professor at the Journalism School at Fudan University in Shanghai, referring to the tendency of local officials to stop the media from reporting disasters in their areas.[6]

In a remarkably frank analysis of the official culture of secrecy, an article in the official Communist Party newspaper, *People's Daily*, noted, "Unfortunately, a long held but outdated conviction among many top public servants dictated that information could also cause possible social panic and disorder. Hence, information was controlled, and this was just what happened at the outset of the SARS outbreak."[7]

Once the Guangdong provincial authorities decided to cover up the disease, the Chinese political structure made it difficult for even the Ministry of Health in Beijing to get information out of Guangdong. The highest ranking official in Guangdong was the provincial Party Secretary, Zhang Dejiang, who was a member of the Politbureau, the highest policy-making body in the Chinese Communist Party. The Guangdong provincial government, including the health authorities, was primarily responsible to him. The Ministry of Health in Beijing had little real authority over the provincial health ministries, and could not compel them to release information. Moreover, once someone as senior as the provincial party secretary, who in the case of Guangdong also happened to be a Politbureau member, had declared that the epidemic was under control, it was impossible for relatively lowly ministers and bureaucrats in Beijing to challenge this. Ultimately, it took Premier Wen Jiabao and President Hu Jintao to unlock the fetters on information about SARS in Guangdong.

Getting information about SARS was also complicated by the fact that disease outbreaks are normally regarded as secret under Chinese laws. It was for this reason that the extent of the HIV/AIDS epidemic in China was not discussed openly until 2002, when the Central authorities decided that the situation was too serious to ignore. Though these laws have been amended before and after SARS, these amendments do not appear to have made it easier for the public to get information about disease outbreaks. Legal and regulatory changes have made it illegal for government officials to hide disease outbreaks from higher authorities. But they have not increased the public's right to know about epidemics.[8]

Besides these considerations, which were unique to the Chinese system, there were other factors at work common to all governments. No country wants to bear the stigma or the economic costs associated with disease. In a world where international trade and investment are the main engines of prosperity, a disease, or any other condition that discourages foreign traders and investors from visiting and doing business, is a kiss of death. Disease is invariably associated with huge business losses. The 1987 plague in India is estimated to have led to business losses of US$2 billion.[9] The British government valiantly tried to persuade a sceptical world that British beef was safe to eat during the BSE crises in the mid-1990s, despite all the evidence to the contrary. And the Guangdong government did its best to pretend to foreign investors, businesspeople and tourists that there was no public health problem in the province and that it was absolutely safe to visit and do business. Guangdong officials admitted as much later, when one of them told a provincial legislator that "they were afraid of the impact of the illness on tourism and investment, because they did not know how to treat the illness."[10]

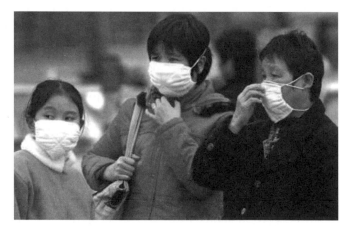

Masked travellers at Guangzhou railway station on February 12, 2003. One of the early signs of public concern about SARS. (photo www.newsgd.com website).

But by February 10, it became obvious that the government would have to say something. There was panic buying of medicine and essential supplies within the province, and fear was beginning to spread to neighbouring provinces. Clearly, continuing to keep quiet would be counterproductive. So on February 11, the provincial government held a press conference acknowledging the presence of the disease and providing some figures on the number of cases, but also announcing that the epidemic was over and that there was no need for anyone to panic.

Huang Qingdao, the head of the Guangdong provincial public health bureau, and other senior health officials provided the press with a fairly detailed account of the origins of the epidemic in December 2002 in the town of Foshan, some 100 kilometres south of Guangzhou, and its progress through other towns in the province until its arrival in Guangzhou. Huang also provided the first official figures for the epidemic: 305 cases, including 105 health care workers, and 5 deaths as of February 9.

The figures he provided were accurate at that point in time. What was wildly off the mark were the government's assurances that there were no more new cases, and that the epidemic was under control. At the time of the press conference, the epidemic was nowhere near under control. It was growing in intensity and there were between 40 and 50 new cases being reported every day. As figures released two months later showed, 688 cases were reported in the province in February, followed by another 364 cases in March and 259 cases in April.

The message underlying the press conference was that this disease was nothing to be worried about: the number of cases was small and the epidemic was dying out. There was no need to panic, and people should get on with their normal lives. To emphasize the point that life should go on as normal, officials stated that a friendly soccer match between China and Brazil scheduled for February 12 would go ahead as planned, and that schools would re-open as usual after the New Year holidays.

The public announcement served its immediate purpose: once the disease was acknowledged officially, the level of panic dropped. On the surface, life in Guangzhou returned to normal. Tough government action against shopkeepers profiting from the panic buying brought prices down, and the people of Guangzhou seemed reassured that the epidemic had died down.

But behind the facade of calm, the Guangdong provincial authorities were grappling with a crisis unlike anything they had faced before. The numbers of cases were increasing, the people who were supposed to treat the disease were falling ill and the hospital system would soon reach breaking point unless the infection was contained. And there were fresh dangers ahead. The Chinese New Year holidays had ended and children were going back to school. If the disease began to spread through the school system, it would be impossible to control.

But a decision had been made at the highest levels of the provincial government that schools and educational institutions would be kept open as a sign that everything was under control in the province, and it was now the responsibility of officials to see that this did not lead to catastrophe. An account of an internal meeting held by the Guangzhou municipal authorities on February 19 reveals the anxieties of government officials as they struggled with the situation.[11] The head of the city's health bureau, Huang Jiongli, warned his colleagues that "if the disease breaks out in schools, it will easily lead to a serious epidemic." The Deputy Mayor of Guangzhou, Chen Zhuanyu, also expressed his concern and said that school principals and the heads of all education units had to take precautions to ensure that the disease did not spread. He warned that with the end of the New Year holidays and the large increase in the number of people travelling to their places of work, the risk that the disease would spread was increasing. "For the moment, unstable factors still exist in society," Chen noted. "Students have gone back to schools, workers have come back to Guangzhou, and disease control and prevention measures are not easy to carry out. If the disease continues to spread, it may lead to another panic outburst, we will face greater pressure."

The head of the Guangzhou health bureau, Huang Jionglie, revealed his true feelings in an off-the-record comment to a journalist: "I cannot tell you whether the situation in Guangzhou is optimistic. I dare not say that today we only have ten new cases, and I cannot guarantee there will not be any tomorrow. We may suddenly discover 100 cases." This anxiety extended to the highest levels of the provincial government. Provincial governor Huang Huaha, in a television interview in June after the epidemic had ended, said, "I could hardly sleep during those days...the epidemic was like a fire and it was a problem of life and death." But the public and the outside world knew nothing of this.

Besides keeping schools and universities open, the Guangdong government also gambled by keeping factories and businesses open throughout the crisis. Guangdong's factories and workshops are manned largely by 10 million migrant workers from poorer provinces. The majority come without their families, and live in dormitories attached to their workplaces. When the epidemic broke, most of these workers had gone back to their homes for the long New Year holiday. They began to return in the second week of February, as the epidemic was reaching its peak. There was a real danger that the poorly ventilated worker dormitories would provide an ideal environment for the explosive spread of the virus, leading to thousands of new cases. But rather than ask factories to delay re-opening, the emphasis of government policy was to keep businesses running as usual.

The provincial government's overriding aim appears to have been to ensure that Guangdong met its GDP growth targets. In an interview broadcast in June by the Chinese state television network CCTV, Zhang Dejiang, the provincial Party Secretary, provided a glimpse of this determination to reach economic growth targets. "We insisted on not suspending class, not stopping producing and ensuring governmental organizations work as usual...All these decisions were based on our scientific knowledge of the epidemic. We found that SARS patients were not infective during the pre-clinical period, so we made this decision. If we made a contrary decision, it would have been impossible to achieve a GDP growth rate of 12.2 percent." [12]

Fortunately, the epidemic did not spread through schools, workplaces and dormitories. But luck appears to have played a part in this. The scientific knowledge on which provincial leaders based their decision was incomplete at the time, and there was no reason to suppose that the epidemic would not spread in educational institutions and workplaces. In Beijing for example, SARS spread in a student dormitory at the Northern Jiaotong University, leading to an exodus of students. And as the outbreak at the Amoy Gardens housing estate in Hong Kong would demonstrate, the SARS virus could spread rapidly in crowded housing.

The decision by the provincial government to disclose only partial truths about SARS did incalculable long-term harm. It kept people in China and the outside world in the dark about the true extent and severity of this new disease, and allowed it to spread beyond the confines of Guangdong province to the wider world.

Take the example of Yu, a businesswoman from Shanxi province. Yu ran a jewellery store in Taiyuan, the provincial capital, and went to Guangdong on February 18 to source supplies for her shop. She returned to Taiyuan on February 23 with what she thought was an ordinary cold and fever. As her symptoms worsened, she went from doctor to doctor looking for a cure. She told the doctors she had been in Guangzhou recently, and asked whether she might have caught the strange pneumonia there had been so many rumours about. The doctors, who had no information about the disease in Guangzhou, laughed off her fears and told her not to worry. Yu described her experience in a letter to the *Beijing Youth Daily* newspaper that reflected the feelings of many other unwitting carriers of the disease: "I have never been able to understand why in an age when it only takes two seconds for information to move from the south to the north of the globe, the top-class hospitals in the provincial capital were unable to obtain more information on the disease, or even a warning about it."[13]

In the first week of March, Yu decided to go to Beijing for medical help. By this time, she had already infected eight family members, including her husband, her parents and five medical staff at the Shanxi Province People's Hospital. Her parents later died of the disease. In Beijing, she saw a doctor at one of the military hospitals, who admitted her to the 302 Army Hospital, which specializes in infectious diseases. As none of the hospital staff were aware that this was a new, highly infectious disease, no special precautions were taken when treating Yu, and more than 10 staff members were infected. This was the first cluster of hospital workers in Beijing to get SARS. Then in April, one of the other patients in the hospital took the disease to Tianjin, a city northeast of Beijing. Yu's uncle in Beijing also fell ill and was admitted to the local You'an Hospital. There he set off a cluster of infections that included one doctor who took the disease to Linhe city in Inner Mongolia. It was through these kinds of incidents that the new disease spread silently through China, shrouded in secrecy until the middle of April, when the problem became so obvious that it was impossible to conceal any longer.

Secrecy also allowed the disease to spread internationally. The health authorities in neighbouring Hong Kong had been alarmed by reports of the new disease and the panic it was causing. But efforts by the Hong Kong Department of Health to find out what was going on from their Guangdong counterparts were met with silence. Later, Hong Kong authorities were told that this was because infectious diseases were a state secret, and could not be disclosed to outsiders. This lack of knowledge about the disease made it possible for a doctor from Guangdong to arrive in a Hong Kong hotel and infect other guests, who would in turn take SARS around the world, passing it on to family members, friends and doctors.

Tragically, the secrecy in Guangdong forced doctors and public health officials in other affected countries to go through the same harsh learning curve as medical workers in Guangdong. By the time the disease escaped to the outside world, doctors in Guangdong knew more about SARS than anyone else. They had worked out guidelines for how patients were to be diagnosed and treated, established effective methods of infection control and put in place public health systems to identify and isolate suspected cases early on so that they would not spread the disease to the wider community. But none of this knowledge was made available to the rest of the world. The Guangdong government saw no reason to disclose it to anyone else. Even provincial health authorities in other parts of China were unaware of the clinical work that had been done in Guangdong until well into the outbreak. Everywhere, health officials and medical workers had to go through the same pattern of trial and error in order to understand the characteristics of this new disease.

The full story of who in the Guangdong provincial government decided to keep the lid on the truth, and whether there were any internal debates over this decision, is not known. The two top provincial leaders, the Party Secretary, Zhang Dejiang, and the Governor, Huang Huahua, have said they informed the Central government and the public about SARS as soon as they were aware of the situation. The Governor maintained that he had sent a message to the State Council in Beijing, the highest body in the Chinese government, on February 7, as soon as he received news about the outbreak. Four days later, the public and the rest of the world were informed through the press conference. What the Governor told the State Council about the scale of the outbreak is unknown. But what his government told the public and the outside world was clearly inadequate.

It was only in April, after the Chinese media was given fairly wide latitude to report on SARS, that media reports critical of the Guangdong provincial government's handling of the disease began to appear. As one commentary said:

> Although SARS was a previously unknown virus, it had been breaking out in Guangdong for as long as three months … why was comprehensive and true information on the SARS virus not promptly given out to the whole country, with the necessary warnings issued? The unfortunate thing is that in the initial stage of the spread of SARS epidemic, until the central authorities adopted decisive measures, information on SARS was not comprehensive … and was even erroneous.[14]

* * *

While the Guangdong provincial government tried to hide the extent of the disease, the provincial public health system responded heroically to the challenge. After being initially overwhelmed by the ferocity of the new illness and the rising tide of patients coming in for treatment, the doctors and public health authorities put together systems of treatment, infection control and contact tracing that were second to none. When a WHO team finally received permission to visit the province in early April, they were impressed by the clinical and public health systems that had been put in place to control SARS, and described Guangdong's efforts as a "model for the rest of China and maybe for the rest of the world."[15] But it took a long process of trial and error before doctors learned enough about the disease to control its spread. Before the SARS epidemic erupted in the city of Guangzhou in early February, the disease had been popping up almost at random at first in one, and then in another of the boom towns in the Pearl River Delta, China's fastest growing region. Each time, the outbreak would attract the attention of the provincial health authorities. But in each instance, it failed to alarm them, because the numbers were small.

The first known case of SARS occurred in November 2002 in the town of Foshan in Guangdong province, an hour's drive south of Guangzhou.[16] The patient was a 46-year-old local government official who was admitted to the Foshan No 1 People's Hospital on November 25 with classic SARS symptoms. He did not infect any of the staff at the hospital, but did spread SARS to five members of his family. How he got the disease remains a mystery. Although SARS would later be linked to a virus that may have passed from civet cats and other animals to humans, at that stage there were no obvious clues.

The disease did not spread in Foshan. But a month later, a 36-year-old restaurant cook, Huang Xingchu, was admitted to hospital in Heyuan, about 100 kilometres north of Guangzhou. Huang worked in a restaurant in Shenzhen, a booming metropolis just across the border from Hong Kong. He had cooked wild animal meat, probably including civet cat, in his restaurant, though it is not clear that this was how he became infected. Huang had begun feeling unwell in early December, and went to his parents' home in Heyuan to recover. After a couple of days at home, his condition worsened, and he was admitted to the local hospital. He had a raging fever, his lungs were congested and he could barely breathe. He had all the symptoms of pneumonia, but this was clearly not a regular form of the disease. It did not clear up with antibiotics, and it was unusual for a pneumonia this severe to attack someone as young and healthy as the chef.

On December 17, as Huang's condition worsened, he was transferred to the Guangzhou military hospital, which had a specialist respiratory diseases department. When he arrived, his lungs were barely functioning, and he was in danger of suffocating to death. He was kept alive on a ventilator for three weeks before recovering. Doctors would have recorded his case as an unusual case of pneumonia and forgotten about it, except for one worrying factor: Huang had left a trail of infection in the hospital in Heyuan, and seven medical workers had come down with the same form of pneumonia. A 41-year-old businessman from Heyuan also contracted the disease after visiting the hospital, and he too was transferred to Guangzhou when local doctors were unable to treat him. Once again, physicians were puzzled by the lack of response to antibiotics and the speed at which the patient's condition deteriorated.

The fact that doctors and nurses were falling ill at the Heyuan hospital alarmed the local hospital authorities. As would be the case in Guangzhou a month later, news that a strange disease was affecting hospital workers spread to the local community and caused general alarm. On January 2, people rushed to pharmacies to buy Western and Chinese medicines, and parents took their children home early from school. The Heyuan city government issued a press release that was carried in the local newspaper assuring people that there had been no deaths, and that there was no virus spreading in the town. The disease that had hit the hospital was attributed to a recent spell of cold weather. As members of the public were buying up large quantities of antibiotics, the public health authorities also urged people not to take medication without the advice of their doctor. The city's education authorities held a meeting with parents to assure them that it was safe to send their children to school. As it happened, this early outbreak did not spread to the community, and after a week, public anxiety had died down and life returned to normal.

On January 2, the Heyuan public health authorities informed the provincial public health authorities about the outbreak. On the same day, the province sent a team of epidemiologists and clinical experts to Heyuan to look into the situation. The experts were puzzled, but there was little alarm as the disease appeared to have died out on its own. As a senior official at the Guangdong provincial health bureau, Feng Liuxiang, recalled, "We sent some experts, and the situation eased soon. We did not take it as an epidemic."[17] Because officials believed the disease had died down, no alert was issued to other towns and cities in the province warning them to be on their guard.

But the disease had not died down. In late December, a patient with similar symptoms turned up in a hospital in Zhongshan, a city some 200 kilometres to the south of Heyuan. Whether the virus was carried to Zhongshan by a sick traveller from Heyuan, or whether there was a local transmission of the virus from animals to humans is not known. The doctors in Zhongshan treated the patient as best they could, but the disease spread, largely among hospital workers who had been treating the patient. By the third week of January, the number of doctors, nurses and hospital assistants falling ill was becoming alarming.

As in Heyuan, reports that a disease was spreading in the hospital system caused public alarm in Zhongshan. People rushed to pharmacies and caused a run on antibiotics. Erythromycin was in particular demand, and the biggest pharmacy chain in the city reported that its stocks of the drug were sold out in four of its eight stores.

The Zhongshan city health authorities alerted the provincial government on January 18 after 28 people, including 13 health care workers, had come down with the disease. The provincial health authorities, who were aware of the earlier outbreak in Heyuan, were alarmed that the disease appeared to be erupting again, and alerted the national Centre for Diseases Control (CDC) in Beijing.

On January 21, a team of experts from Beijing and Guanghzou arrived in Zhongshan to investigate the outbreak and devise a strategy to prevent its spread. The most prominent member of the team was Zhong Nanshan, the 67-year-old head of the Guangdong Institute for Respiratory Diseases. A slim, ascetic-looking man who would become a pivotal figure in China's struggle against SARS, Zhong was widely respected for his medical knowledge, his devotion to his patients and his habit of speaking his mind.

In the weeks ahead, he was an often lonely voice urging the government to seek international assistance to find the cause of the disease and speaking out against political interference in the fight against SARS. The son of an eminent professor of paediatrics in Guangzhou, Zhong would later say that his dogged belief that policy should be based on scientific fact rather than political expedience reflected what he had learned from his father: "My father never exaggerated anything. He spoke of the facts and his experiments."[18]

Zhong took on the political authorities on several occasions. When government officials in first Guangdong and later in Beijing declared that the disease was under control, Zhong flatly contradicted them. At a public forum in Beijing, he said it was premature to say the disease was under control. "How can you bring the disease under control when you don't know its cause?" he asked. [19]

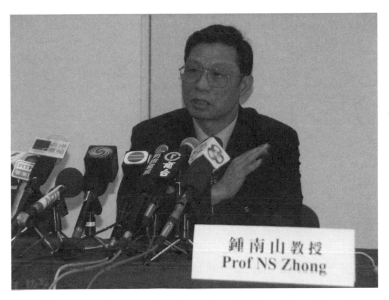

Zhong Nanshan, a key figure in the fight against SARS in China, pictured here at a press conference in Hong Kong. (courtesy The University of Hong Kong)

Zhong had earlier disputed the official wisdom from Beijing that the cause of SARS was not a new coronavirus, but chlamydia, a bacteria that can be easily cured by antibiotics. He pointed out that antibiotics had proven to be of no use in treating SARS and warned against the treatment regime that the Central authorities had proposed.

As a member of the Chinese Academy of Sciences, and a respected figure in China's medical and scientific establishment, Zhong could get away with being outspoken. And as opinion shifted towards greater openness at the highest level of the Chinese government in late April, his position was vindicated and he was officially hailed as one of the heroes of China's fight against SARS.

Zhong had first become aware of the new disease in late December when he saw one of the two patients from Heyuan who had been transferred to Guangzhou. It was clear to him that this was no ordinary pneumonia. The most unusual clinical feature was the state of the patient's lungs. "His lungs were hard," Zhong recalled in an interview broadcast over China's CCTV television network. "Normally lungs are like a rubber ball which can expand or shrink as air is pumped in or taken out. Yet this patient's lungs were like plastic, without any elasticity." X-rays of the patient's chest showed an unusual opaque pattern, somewhat like ground glass.

Zhong was alarmed by the trail of infection that the patient from Heyuan had set off in his family and among hospital workers, and discussed his concerns with the Guangdong health authorities. The emergence of a new cluster of disease in Zhongshan, 200 kilometres away from the earlier outbreak, seemed to confirm his fears that this was a disease that was not only contagious, but was also spreading across the Pearl River Delta.

Zhong Nanshan and the team from Beijing worked through the night of January 21 reviewing the cases in Zhongshan city and produced the first description of the new disease, its symptoms and possible methods of treatment. They named the disease "atypical pneumonia," or *feidian* in Chinese, a name that would stick until the WHO named it SARS more than six weeks later. The data that had been gathered from the cases in Heyuan as well as the new evidence from Zhongshan pointed to an unusual pneumonia possibly caused by a virus. Since tests on patients had not revealed the presence of any of the common viruses, this was most likely to be a virus of unknown origin. From the pattern of infection, researchers also concluded that the disease was spread through respiratory droplets.

The five-page report Zhong and his colleagues produced, known as the No 2 Report, described the basic clinical features of the disease and set out a range of treatment options that included both Chinese and Western medical techniques. It suggested treatment with corticosteroids and artificial respirators for critically ill patients, specified that patients should be quarantined and emphasized the importance of good ventilation and disinfection to prevent the disease spreading in hospitals. It also set out the infection control measures that hospital staff needed to take to stop the spread of the disease, including the wearing of masks and frequent hand washing.

The report was handed over to the provincial health authorities on January 23. By the end of the month, its main recommendations were distributed to major hospitals in Guangzhou. This document would have been an invaluable resource for the international community once SARS escaped into the wider world. But the Guangdong provincial authorities took no steps to share it with other countries struggling with the disease.

The big worry at the end of January was that the epidemic would spread from the smaller towns and cities to the provincial capital Guangzhou, a crowded metropolis of around 9 million people. Starting from the middle of December, serious cases from provincial towns had been transferred to the better-equipped hospitals in Guangzhou. By the middle of January, the first signs that the disease was spreading in the

广东省卫生厅办公室文件

粤卫办〔2003〕2号

关于印发省专家组关于中山市不明原因
肺炎调查报告的通知

各地级以上市卫生局、省直、部属驻穗及厅直属各医疗卫生单位:

近期，我省广州、深圳、佛山、河源、中山等地先后发生人数不等的"不明原因肺炎"(非典型肺炎)病人。我厅派出专家组到河源市、中山市等地进行了调查，现将《省专家组关于中山市不明原因肺炎调查报告》(以下简称《调查报告》)印发给你们，并提出如下几点意见，请认真贯彻执行:

一、各市卫生行政部门、各级医疗卫生机构要高度重视，组织医疗卫生人员认真学习《调查报告》，特别是学习和掌握其中的"治疗原则"及"预防措施"。今后凡发现有类似病人，要严加

- 1 -

观察和诊治。

二、各级医疗机构要加强 ICU 建设和管理，一旦发现非典型肺炎类似病例，要及时按照其治疗原则正确隔离救治病人，严防医治不当引致死亡的发生。同时要及时将疫情报告当地疾病预防控制机构，以采取有效预防措施，防止疫情的扩散蔓延。

三、各地要加强正面宣传教育，普及呼吸道感染疾病的防治知识，切实提高群众自我保健意识和能力，减少疾病发生，避免造成不良的社会影响。

附件: 省专家组关于中山市非典型肺炎调查报告

二〇〇三年二月二十三日

The January 23 document issued by the Guangdong provincial health authorities. This was the first official document issued by the provincial health authorities about SARS. Some hospitals did not receive it until nearly two weeks later. (This document is available on the Canadian Broadcasting Corporation website, *www.cbc.ca/disclosure.*)

hospital system appeared. The Guangdong provincial hospital for traditional Chinese medicine was the first to be hit. It had begun receiving patients from Zhongshan on January 14. The disease was still unknown at that time and hospital staff did not take any particular precautions when treating patients. By January 28, seven staff members had come down with fever and a dry cough and chest X-rays showed shadows on their lungs.

On January 30, the Guangdong public health bureau received reports from other hospitals that the number of pneumonia patients they were receiving was rising. The next day, the authorities decided to centralize treatment and ordered that all pneumonia patients be transferred to one of seven designated hospitals. Zhong Nanshan took the most serious cases to the Institute for Respiratory Diseases, attached to the Guangzhou University Medical School. The No 2 Report was circulated to hospitals, and staff members were asked to implement infection control measures.

But nothing could prepare medical workers for the storm that was to hit them during the first week of February when Zhou Zuofeng, the man described earlier as the "poison king," triggered an epidemic in three Guangzhou hospitals. Zhou was what is loosely described as a "super-spreader" — a patient who spreads infection to a disproportionately large number of other people.

At the start of the epidemic, the average SARS patient spread the infection to between two and three new people. This is not a particularly high rate of transmission, and taken alone these numbers would not have caused the epidemic to spread so rapidly. But there were a handful of people around the world who managed to infect a disproportionately large number of other people, creating explosions of disease. Researchers refer to these as super-spreading events, reflecting the fact that it is not merely the individuals involved who are responsible for the phenomenon, but also a series of other factors including the effectiveness of the infection control measures adopted, environmental factors and a number of other variables that are still not fully understood.

The trail of infection triggered by Zhou Zoufeng in the Guangzhou hospital system was the first of these super-spreading events. Besides triggering the epidemic in Guangzhou, this event would also result in the transfer of the disease to Hong Kong, where it would travel to the rest of the world via another super-spreading event. The epidemic in Hong Kong was set off by a doctor from Guangzhou who had contracted the disease at the Second Affiliated Hospital, the first hospital to which Zhou was admitted.

When Zhou arrived at the No 3 Affiliated Hospital, he was delirious, coughing up a bloody phlegm, and it seemed unlikely he would survive long. Doctors in the emergency room decided he had to be put on a mechanical ventilator if he was to have any chance of survival. This involved opening his mouth, clearing out the accumulated phlegm, moving the patient's tongue out of the way and then inserting the tube directly into the airway. In Zhou's case, it took a nerve-wracking two hours for this relatively simple procedure to the completed.[20]

Though he was sedated, Zhou, a large, heavy-set man, still managed to thrash around, making it impossible to get a tube into his mouth. One group of doctors and nurses held down his arms, legs and head, while others tried to insert the tube. Each time they began to insert the tube, there was an eruption of blood-tinged mucous. It splashed on to the floor, the equipment and the faces and gowns of the medical staff. They knew the mucous was highly infectious, and in the normal course of things, they would have cleaned themselves up as quickly as possible. But with a critically ill patient kicking and heaving around, a tube half-inserted into his windpipe and mucous and blood spurting out, there was no way any of them could leave. For what seemed like an eternity they battled with the barely conscious patient, clearing his airways of mucous, keeping his lungs and heart going, trying to keep his head still enough so that the tube could be guided in without damaging his teeth, tongue or vocal chords and attempting to keep out of the way of the virus-laden eruptions. By the time the procedure was completed, Zhou had calmed down, and the ventilator was pumping oxygen to his lungs. But the medical workers were exhausted and terrified that they too might catch his disease.

Two days later, doctors who had helped intubate Zhou started falling ill with fever, chills and headaches. Their chest X-rays revealed shadows on their lungs. Within a week of Zhou's admission, 20 doctors and medical workers who had been involved in treating him had been infected.

As health care workers dealing with SARS around the world would discover in the weeks and months ahead, treating this disease needed more than sound medical skills. It required courage. Each time doctors, nurses or assistants went near a patient, they knew they were risking their lives. Health care workers took to wearing four and five layers of masks, gloves and protective outer garments. But all these layers of protection seemed to do was add to their discomfort. Even simple tasks became that much more difficult when swathed in the extra layers of garments. And in the warmth of Guangdong, the protective masks and garments made the medical workers sweat constantly, especially after hospitals began to switch off central air conditioning systems in case the virus was being transmitted through air-conditioning vents. Medical workers also knew that they were putting their families in danger each time they went home from the hospital.

The experience at the No 8 People's Hospital in Guangzhou was typical of the stresses undergone by medical staff in the early stages of the epidemic. "We received our first five patients on February 2," recalled Tang Xiaoping, the head of the hospital. "They all had a high fever, cough and difficulty in breathing. The number gradually increased. We had 30 coming in on February 6, 30 on February 8, and by February 12 we had over 150."[21]

The No 8 hospital is a relatively small medical facility with around 200 medical staff. Staff members, working 24-hour shifts, were overwhelmed by the sudden increase in the number of critically ill patients they were treating. "At that time, most of the doctors and nurses had been working from February 2 onwards non stop for 10 days. They worked for more than 10 hours a day. On the 12th and 13th of February, 4 medical workers fainted in the sick wards ... but after a short break they went on working," said Tang Xiaoping.

Though the provincial health authorities had issued guidelines on the wearing of masks and infection control, medical staff were unused to taking these kinds of precautionary measures and many did not. "We didn't wear masks or goggles then because we didn't have any experience of the disease ... we had never encountered such a highly infectious disease even though I have been treating infectious diseases for more than ten years," said Tang. Medical staff then took to wearing as many as 12 layers of surgical masks. But they were still coming down with the disease. It took a few days for them to realize that they were being infected through the tissues of the eyes. Goggles were then added to the list of protective equipment.

Despite these precautions, by February 13, 11 days after the first patients were admitted, medical staff at the No 8 People's Hospital began to fall ill. "From the 13th to the 19th, 20 medical workers fell ill. As the situation got more and more serious, I thought the hospital might have to be closed off, and the pressure on me was almost unendurable," recalled Tang.

Zhang Jihui, a senior nurse at the No 1 People's Hospital in Guangzhou, kept a diary of her experiences during the SARS outbreak that was excerpted in Guangzhou newspapers. The No 1 hospital had been designated to receive critically ill medical personnel, and received its first patient on February 17. On February 19, Zhang noted: "Just two days, and all the nurses have the same feeling — exhausted physically and psychologically. Every day the doctors keep patrolling the sick wards and adjust the treatment according to the patients' situation. And the nurses ceaselessly carry out the order of the doctors. As they are all dressed in many layers of clothes: work clothes, isolation suits, thick surgical masks, shuttling back and forth in the sick wards makes them drenched."[22]

A day later Zhang wrote: "Another group of infected medical staff transferred here. This means we will be busier, and our duty hours will be extended ... almost everyone's feet are swollen. The hospital gives us wonderful food every day, but no one can eat ... our only wish is to sleep, even if only a nap of 10 minutes in the office." Working conditions were similar in other hospitals throughout the city as medical staff toiled away with a simple heroism under conditions in which they knew they were risking their lives.

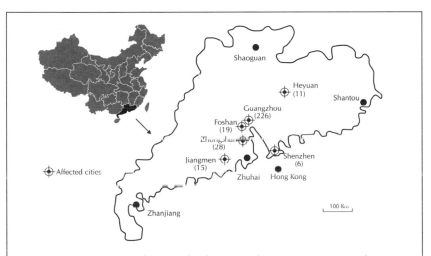

The geographic distribution of SARS outbreak in Guangdong Nov 16, 2002, to Feb 9, 2003. Number of cases are shown in brackets. Approximate dates of the onset of the outbreaks for each city were Foshan, Nov 16, 2002; Heyuan, Dec 17, 2002; Zhongshan, Dec 26, 2003; Guangzhou, Jan 31, 2003; Jiangmen, Jan 10, 2003; Shenzhen, Jan 15, 2003.

Map of Guangdong province showing how the disease spread. Reprinted with permission from Elsevier (*The Lancet* vol. 362, 2003 p. 354)

The biggest handicap in those early weeks was the lack of knowledge about the disease. Zhong Nanshan's No 2 Report had set out basic information about the disease, but there were still many gaps. Modern evidence-based medicine relies on complex scientific studies to establish the cause of a disease, method of transmission, incubation period, symptoms and treatment. In the case of a new disease, researchers are forced to start from scratch. And when the disease causes a public health emergency, as was the case with SARS, it creates enormous pressure for researchers to come up with rapid answers to questions that normally take years to resolve.

Zhong Nanshan was appointed by the Guangdong provincial authorities to head a small group of experts to study the disease and come up with an effective method of controlling it. "The biggest challenge I had to face was probably ignorance about the disease. We didn't know where to start, we had no clear diagnosis, and no effective cure," recalled Zhong.[23] He began by meticulously recording the symptoms of every patient admitted to hospital and the details of how he or she might have got the disease. He also noted the changes that occurred as the disease progressed, particularly the way the lungs deteriorated, as well as the response to different kinds of treatment. Autopsies and examination of the lung tissue of patients showed the extraordinary damage caused by the disease. The virus destroyed the alveoli, the tiny sacs that line the inside of the lungs and allow oxygen to pass into the blood stream and carbon dioxide to pass out. The delicate membranes that allow this exchange of gases to occur were scarred, and instead of air, the lungs were filled with a mixture of blood and dead cells.

Since the agent causing this damage was unknown, Zhong developed a treatment to give the lungs as much protection as possible. In the early stages of the disease, as the patches on a patient's lungs increased, the first step was to increase the oxygen flow to the lungs through an oxygen mask using CPAP, or continuous positive airway pressure. This is a method of oxygen delivery does not require the introduction of a tube into the airways, and Zhong found that in many patients, early use of oxygen masks prevented deterioration in the lungs. If X-rays showed that the disease was progressing to a more severe stage, then Zhong advocated the use of corticosteroids, which are known to reduce inflammation in lung tissue. Traditional Chinese medicines were also used to reduce fever and lung congestion.

Corticosteroids were later used by doctors across the world, from Beijing to Toronto, but their use became controversial after patients in China and Hong Kong developed avascular necrosis, a crippling bone disease, as a side effect of the steroids. In Guangzhou, where Zhong supervised treatment and specified the precise dosage of steroids and the duration for which they were to be used, three percent of patients developed bone problems. In Beijing, where corticosteroids were used more liberally, as many as 33 percent of recovered SARS patients are thought to have developed avascular necrosis. Zhong later said that he should have been clearer as to the optimum dosage of steroids for the benefit of doctors elsewhere who followed his treatment regime.[24]

One of the earliest challenges was to define the new disease in a way that would allow doctors to distinguish between SARS patients and those with other forms of pneumonia and influenza. This was particularly difficult in the case of SARS, where there were no distinctive symptoms in the early stages of the disease. The fever, dry cough, body aches and occasional breathlessness that SARS patients first exhibited were symptoms associated with a variety of diseases. Since the disease was new and no one knew what was causing it, there were no blood tests or any other method of detecting SARS patients before they developed full symptoms. But doctors could not afford to wait until the full symptoms developed before beginning to treat patients. The challenge was to describe the disease in such a way that SARS cases would not be missed, but not to define it so widely that every patient with a fever or cough would be treated as a potential SARS case. The choice medical researchers had to make was between defining the disease so narrowly that SARS cases who did not have all of the symptoms would be missed, or defining it so widely that people with other diseases would be seen as potential SARS cases.

The crucial feature of SARS appeared to be that you could only get the disease after close contact with a patient. Therefore, a history of contact with a known SARS patient within the past 20 days became an important element of the case definition. A fever above 38°C, a dry cough and body aches, lack of response to antibiotics and chest X-rays that showed a characteristic pattern were laid down as the other elements to look for when diagnosing SARS cases. In the end, this definition was not perfect: a large number of SARS patients in Guangdong appear to have developed the disease without having been in close contact with a SARS patient. Patients with influenza and other diseases with SARS-like symptoms often found themselves caught in the SARS net. But as an initial working definition, this helped doctors and public health workers to have a fairly clear idea of what they were looking for.

But since this case definition was not public knowledge outside of the Guangdong hospital system, six weeks later in mid-March, once SARS had reached the outside world, WHO officials would have to go through the same process to come up with a definition of the disease.

Because WHO officials in Geneva had far less knowledge of the disease and its symptoms than Guangdong health officials, their definition was necessarily broader and less specific. It was only in early April, when WHO teams were finally allowed into Guangdong, that they found that much of the work they had struggled to do had already been done.

The experience gained in February 2003, when the epidemic in Guangzhou was at its peak, was distilled down to five principles for treating and containing the disease: early discovery of cases, early reporting of cases, early isolation of cases, careful use of steroids and careful use of artificial ventilation. On March 9, a few days before SARS received international attention, the Guangdong health authorities issued a definitive document entitled, "Work Instruction on the Treatment of Atypical Pneumonia for Hospitals in Guangdong." This was an expanded version of the No 2 Report issued at the end of January and took into account the experience that had been gained since then. This definitive document set out the protocol for diagnosis and treatment of SARS. But once again, the policy of official silence meant that the rest of the world was deprived of this information. Doctors in Hong Kong, Singapore, Vietnam and Canada had to go through the same process of trial and error to rediscover what their counterparts in Guangdong already knew.

Guidelines were also laid down to prevent the disease from spreading in public places such as restaurants, schools and workplaces and on public transport. A crucial element in Guangdong's strategy to stop the disease from spreading was a system of meticulous contact tracing: anyone who came down with the disease was asked to list all of the people with whom he or she had been in close contact in the three weeks before falling ill. These people were then interviewed, and those suspected of having caught the disease were quarantined or hospitalized to see that they did not spread it any further. By catching potential SARS cases early, and getting them to hospital quickly, the chain of transmission was gradually broken.

February was the peak of the epidemic in Guangdong. By March, doctors and public health authorities knew enough about the disease to be able to contain its spread both among the general public and in the hospital system. But the storm that had begun in the province was now about to sweep through the rest of China.

* * *

Of all the world cities affected by SARS, Beijing was hit the hardest. Of the 8098 SARS cases reported across the world, 2521, more than a quarter, occurred in this city alone. And of all the outbreaks in the world, this one was the most preventable. It was also the most politically charged, threatening the stability of the newly appointed Chinese leadership.

The period between the autumn of 2002, when the first cases of SARS emerged in Guangdong, and the spring of 2003, when outbreaks of the disease occurred in China and around the world, was also a pivotal period in Chinese politics. The generation of Communist Party leaders that had led China during the 1990s was handing over power to a new generation. Jiang Zemin, who had led China for more than a decade, was in the process of transferring power to Hu Jintao, one of his vice-presidents. But there was uncertainty about how much power he would hand over to his successor, and how much he would retain himself. In November 2002, some of this uncertainty ended when Jiang Zemin handed over one of his key positions, as General Secretary of the Communist Party, to Hu Jintao, and also stepped down from the Party's key decision making body, the Politbureau.

But Jiang still held two important official positions as President of China and head of the Chinese military. Would he hand these positions over as well, or would it be an extended transition of power? These questions would be resolved at the meeting of the National People's Congress in March 2003, when decisions regarding the leadership of the government, as opposed to the Party, would be unveiled.

All of the energy of the Party and the governmental machinery was focused on ensuring that any political changes in the offing would go smoothly. Stability had to be maintained during this period, and no false note could be struck in the run-up to the National People's Congress. If anything went wrong in the carefully orchestrated political transition, China's ambitious programme of modernization would be placed at risk. As far as the government was concerned, news of disease or other disasters that could lead to public unrest and political uncertainty would certainly not be allowed to mar the smoothness of the transition.[25]

It was in this politically charged period, when the whole of China was focused on who the country's new leaders would be, that the SARS virus crept into Beijing. And by a quirk of history, the dates on which the first SARS cases arrived in Beijing coincided with the key dates on which the transfer of power occurred. March 5, when the National People's Congress began the two-week meeting at which the new leadership would be announced, was also the day that Beijing received its first SARS case: Yu, the businesswoman from Shanxi who had contracted the disease during a visit to Guangdong. On March 15, Hu

Jintao was formally appointed President by the Congress. This was the same day that a second patient, a 72-year-old man who had contracted SARS while on a visit to Hong Kong, was taken to a hospital in Beijing. He was the first super-spreader in the capital and infected at least 59 other people with the disease. Those infected by him would then cause outbreaks in Inner Mongolia and Taiwan.

With everyone's attention on the two men who would lead the country, President Hu Jintao and Premier Wen Jiabao, it is unlikely that anyone was paying attention to two sick people admitted to the city's hospitals. But within a month, the chain of events triggered by these two cases would snowball into an epidemic that challenged the survival of the new leadership.

The SARS epidemic in Beijing began in March and reached its peak in the second half of April, when there were more than 100 cases a day admitted to hospitals. As in Guangdong, the disease was transmitted by early cases in the hospitals to health care workers and other patients before seeping out into the community. And as in Guangdong, the first response to the outbreak was to keep it hidden and deny that there was any problem so that "social stability" would not be affected.

As the experience of Guangdong showed, hiding an epidemic of this magnitude allowed it to spread through lack of knowledge. Doctors and nurses in Beijing knew nothing about the experience of their colleagues in Guangdong in fighting SARS. All they knew was that there had been an outbreak of atypical pneumonia that had been brought under control by the middle of February. They were unaware of how infectious it was or how easily it spread in hospitals. And crucially, they were not watching out for possible cases of SARS because the epidemic was thought to have died out in Guangdong.

The description of the disease in Guangdong as "atypical pneumonia" also contributed to a certain complacency in Beijing. Atypical pneumonia is a broad term that covers a variety of diseases. In many cases, atypical pneumonia can be milder than the so-called typical community-acquired pneumonia caused by the *pneumoccocus* bacteria. "Many clinical doctors did not believe that atypical pneumonia can be that serious and were therefore slow to respond," commented Cai Boqiang, head of the respiratory diseases department at one of Beijing's main teaching hospitals.[26] This complacency was compounded by the announcement in late February by the Chinese Centre for Diseases Control (CDC) that the epidemic in Guangdong was caused by chlamydia, a bacteria that is easily treatable with antibiotics.

By the middle of March, medical workers who treated the first few cases in Beijing were going through the same learning process that their colleagues in Guangdong had experienced. Despite the official silence, rumours about the disease had begun to spread through internet chat rooms and bulletin boards. On March 26, the government briefly acknowledged that SARS existed in Beijing: a report issued by the official Xinhua news agency quoted city health officials as saying that there were a few cases that had been "imported" from other parts of the country, but that the disease was not spreading locally.

As SARS spread across the world, and the evidence pointed to the epidemic having originated in China, international pressure on the Chinese authorities to reveal more about the disease grew. In Beijing, the authorities responded by stating that the city had a small number of cases that were not spreading locally. On April 3, China's Health Minister, Zhang Wenkang, declared at a televised press conference that Beijing had 12 cases of SARS, of whom three had died, but emphasized that the disease was well under control. "Beijing has learned lessons from Guangdong and has effectively controlled its imported cases and a few cases caused by these imported cases. Therefore it hasn't spread out into society."[27]

At the time the Health Minister was delivering these assurances, there were well over 100 cases in Beijing, and the numbers were rising steadily. The new leadership was clearly worried about the disease, and was itself trying to understand the severity of the problem. On April 2, the situation was discussed by the State Council Executive Committee, a high-level ministerial body headed by Premier Wen Jiabao. A *Xinhua* report of the meeting said that committee members were told that SARS had "already been brought under effective control." But if SARS had indeed been brought under control, it would not have been discussed at this level of government. The new leaders were themselves apparently struggling to understand the full magnitude of the crisis. According to a report in *The Washington Post*, Premier Wen was finding it difficult to get accurate information about how many cases there were in Beijing. [28]

A major obstacle to gathering information appears to have been that most of the cases at the time were in military hospitals, and while the military was reporting these cases to its own chain of command, this information was not being reported to the civilian authorities. The first two SARS cases in Beijing, the businesswoman from Shanxi and the 72-year-old man who brought the disease from Hong Kong, had both been admitted to military hospitals where they set off clusters of infection among doctors and nurses. The Beijing city authorities were also concealing the numbers of cases in their own hospitals from the Central authorities in case they were taken to task for allowing the disease to spread in the capital. *The Washington Post* quoted one Western ambassador in Beijing as saying, "It was as if an epidemic raged in Washington but was kept secret from the White House."[29]

The lid on the SARS story was thrown open by an unlikely whistle-blower: a 72-year-old retired military surgeon. Jiang Yanyong had joined the People's Liberation Army (PLA) in 1954, and retired as head of surgery at the 301 Hospital, the main military hospital in Beijing. At the time of the SARS outbreak, he saw patients once a week at the 301 Hospital and performed the occasional surgery.

He first became aware of the extent of the SARS epidemic when an old friend and fellow doctor had to have surgery for lung cancer at the end of March. When he was admitted for surgery, the patient was found to have a high fever and unusual patches on his lungs. It turned out that he had SARS. When Jiang telephoned the No 309 PLA Hospital to enquire about his friend, he was told that the hospital had 40 cases of SARS, with six deaths. The next day, he was told the number of cases had risen to 60. The No 302 Hospital had 40 cases, he learned.[30]

On April 3, he watched Health Minister Zhang Wenkang declare on television that there were only 12 SARS cases in Beijing. Jiang Yanyong was outraged by this attempt to downplay a disease that he knew was spreading in Beijing.

The retired surgeon did an unusual thing. He wrote a letter accusing the minister of covering up the true extent of the SARS outbreak in Beijing and emailed it to two television stations: the main state broadcaster CCTV, and Hong Kong-based broadcaster Phoenix TV. Jiang's letter said that he "couldn't believe what he was hearing" when the Health Minister said there were only 12 SARS cases in the city. Doctors and nurses at the military hospitals in Beijing were outraged as well, he added. Health Minister Zhang was a fellow medical professional, but Jiang wrote that he had "abandoned his fundamental sense of moral integrity as a doctor."[31]

Jiang also confirmed in his letter that the military hospital system had received its first SARS cases in early March at the time of the opening of the National People's Congress. He said that the civilian authorities at the Ministry of Health had known about these cases, but told hospital authorities not to publicize the cases in order to "ensure stability" during the congress.

Jiang Yanyong's revelations were not reported immediately by the media in China, but his letter was picked up by *Time* magazine, which brought it to international attention. The *Time* report appeared on the internet, allowing people in China to read it as well. Despite a brief period of uncertainty about what would happen to him, Jiang became something of a media celebrity, and as news reporting about SARS loosened up, even government publications like *China Daily* were writing glowing articles about his courage.

After Jiang's revelations were made public, the government's attempts to cover up the scale of the epidemic were looking increasingly thin. People in Beijing took to wearing masks, and foreign visitors began to put off travel to China. The death due to SARS of a visiting International Labour Organization representative, Pekka Aro, focused international attention on the situation in Beijing. A WHO team that arrived in the city was greeted with a farcical attempt to bundle patients out of two military hospitals that the team planned to inspect and send them to a third hospital. WHO officials in Beijing had by now abandoned their customary diplomatic reticence and were openly accusing the authorities of concealing the true number of SARS cases. On April 16, when the official figures indicated there were only 37 cases in the capital, Alan Schnur, a senior official at the WHO's Beijing office, told journalists that he believed there were between 100 and 200 cases in the capital.[32]

While bureaucrats and lower-level ministers were continuing to maintain that Beijing was a perfectly safe city and that there was no epidemic, the new leadership of President Hu and Premier Wen was sending a very different message. At a national SARS prevention meeting on April 16, Wen described the situation as "extremely grave." He also made it clear that the government's ability to control SARS would be crucial to achieving China's economic reform and modernization programme. "The situation of reform, development and stability, the nation's interests and China's image in the international community" were all at stake, he said.[33] A day later, on April 17, Hu called a meeting of the Communist Party's highest body, the Politbureau, at which he apparently emphasized the gravity of the situation and stressed the need for greater transparency from officials.

The first results of this new policy of acknowledging the problem and fighting it openly became clear two days later on April 19. Journalists in Beijing who were called to a press conference with the Health Minster, Zhang Wenkang, were surprised to find his deputy, Gao Qiang, addressing them. Equally surprising were the figures that he delivered: instead of 39 cases, as stated earlier, the capital now had 339 cases, including 18 deaths. In addition, there were another 402 suspected cases of SARS in Beijing. Gao went on to announce the extent to which the disease was spreading across China: Shanxi province had 108 cases, Inner Mongolia had 25, Guangxi had 12, Fujian had 3 and Shanghai had 2.

Later in the day, it became clear why the Health Minister had not turned up in person to announce these figures. A terse government announcement stated that he and the Mayor of Beijing, Meng Xuenong, had been sacked for their lack of transparency about the disease.

After being hidden for months, first in Guangdong and then in Beijing, SARS was now out in the open. All of the efforts of the Chinese government were focused on controlling the epidemic. In Beijing, the immediate focus was on stopping the spread of the disease by limiting the movement of people, detecting cases early on and getting patients to hospital quickly. Schools and universities were shut, and tough quarantine regulations were introduced, giving the authorities the power to isolate hospitals, factories, hotels, restaurants, offices and residential buildings and any other locations where there was a danger that the disease would spread to large numbers of people. By April 26, 4000 people who had been in contact with SARS patients had been quarantined, university students were asked not to leave their campuses, and cinemas, theatres, internet cafes and other places of entertainment where people might gather were shut down. The treatment of SARS patients was streamlined, with six hospitals designated to receive SARS patients.

The speed and scale on which China can operate once mobilized was illustrated by its amazing feat in constructing a fully operational, 1000-bed SARS hospital at a cost of US$170 million within a week on the outskirts of Beijing. Construction of the hospital began on April 26, near the site of a former sanatorium, and it was opened to the first patients on May 2. Seven thousand workers completed the buildings in six days and seven nights using prefabricated materials. One thousand two hundred military doctors, nurses and assistants were brought into Beijing from all over China to staff the well-equipped facility. By the time the hospital discharged its last patient on June 21, it had treated 680 patients, of whom only eight had died.

Beijing, as the capital city, was given all the resources it needed to fight SARS, and there was little doubt that it would succeed. The real danger was that SARS would explode in China's rural areas and poorer provinces, which did not have either the medical or the financial resources to fight the epidemic. If SARS spread through China's vast rural areas, it would become almost impossible to control. And if SARS became permanently established in rural China, then it was only a matter of time before it reappeared in cities, and from there travelled to the outside world.

By April, SARS had already appeared in some of China's poorest provinces, including Inner Mongolia, Guanxi and Hebei. With workplaces and construction sites in Beijing closed, there were worries that migrant workers would leave the city and return to the poorer provinces they came from, bringing SARS with them. According to some estimates, over 2 million workers had left Guangdong and Beijing and returned to their home provinces. Across the country, local government officials were mobilized to check on travellers with fever or any other SARS symptoms, and money was poured into upgrading badly under-funded epidemic monitoring systems. Fortunately, these measures proved sufficient to prevent SARS from spreading into China's poorer provinces. Of the 5327 cases reported in China, 4033 were from the cities of Beijing and Guangzhou. Small clusters of infection were also reported in 22 other provinces, but only amounted to 1294 cases.

SARS had been a baptism by fire for the new Chinese leadership. Because the disease had been largely confined to two major cities with well-developed health systems, the government had been able to focus all its attention on stamping out the disease and had done so successfully. But this success came at a cost. Over 5300 people had been infected and 349 had died. Had there been greater openness about the disease, those who were at risk might have taken precautions to avoid infection. Once the Central government acknowledged the gravity of the situation, the need for openness and transparency were widely trumpeted in the media and in speeches by the new leaders.

For a while, the media did enjoy an unusual degree of latitude in reporting on SARS and on official attempts to hide it in the early stages of the epidemic. But old ways seemed to reassert themselves fairly quickly. When a case of SARS occurred in early 2004 in Guangdong, it was reported by the *Southern Metropolitan Daily* newspaper. But the provincial authorities, who had not made an official announcement about the case, expressed their displeasure that it had been reported without prior authorization from the government. Zeng Wenqiong, the journalist who wrote the story, was prevented from further reporting on SARS and assigned to other duties on the newspaper. The lesson that a free flow of information can help prevent the spread of disease had not yet been learned.

3

HONG KONG

THE police vans came a little before 6 a.m. and drove right up to the entrance of the apartment building. As the sun's first light broke through the tightly packed tower blocks of eastern Kowloon, policemen tumbled out and rapidly erected makeshift barricades at the entrance to Block E of Amoy Gardens, one of 19 blocks in a typical Hong Kong middle income housing development.

Besides the normal equipment carried by the Hong Kong policeman — handcuffs, service revolver and walkie talkie — each officer had strapped around his nose and mouth an N95 mask with a filter fine enough to trap microbial particles. With the policemen came health officials and social workers, gowned and masked like surgeons, covered from head to toe in white protective covering, carrying a letter for each of the 254 flats in the block.

As police guarded the entrance, health officials went from floor to floor, knocking on each door and handing the startled, sleepy householders a government order stating that they would not be able to step out of their apartments for the next ten days. Neither would anyone be able to visit them. They would be brought three cooked meals a day, their pets would be fed as well, and daily necessities would be brought to them.

Many were angry. How would they go to work? Who was going to take the dog for a walk? Why should the government lock them up in their own houses? But most were resigned to their fate. For days now, SARS had been raging through Amoy Gardens. In less than a week, 213 cases had been reported among the residents of the complex, a third of all the cases in Hong Kong. And more than half of these had come from Block E. Many residents had already fled, moving in with friends and relatives or checking into hotels. There was a killer loose in the building, and they wanted to get as far away as possible.

But there was worse to come. The Hong Kong health authorities discovered it was impossible to investigate the cause of the outbreak while residents were still in their homes. They would have to be moved out. So the next night, clutching bags of belongings and blinking under the glare of television cameras, residents were taken like refugees to an isolated holiday camp where they were quarantined for two weeks.

For the rest of Hong Kong, those televised images of masked and gowned health workers and policemen shepherding the Amoy Gardens residents on to buses to be driven off into quarantine seemed to symbolize the depths to which their city had plunged.

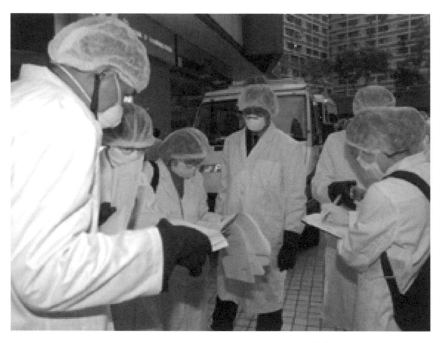

Health workers prepare to enter Block E, Amoy Gardens and serve isolation orders on the tenants. (Courtesy: Government Information Services, HKSAR)

Amoy Gardens epitomized the disaster that had hit Hong Kong. Like the apartment complex, Hong Kong itself was in the grips of a stealthy killer, invisible, cunning, seemingly able to strike at will, and against whom there seemed to be no defence. In a matter of weeks, a brash, vibrant city of 6 million had been reduced by the fear of disease to a ghost of its former self. Surgical masks, rarely seen outside of hospital operating theatres, suddenly became an essential item of daily wear. Businesses made it compulsory for their employees to wear masks at work and everyone from high-flying investment bankers to shop assistants conducted their daily activities wearing surgical masks.

Hong Kong was under virtual quarantine. Its showpiece airport with airy vaulted ceilings, designed by the British architect Sir Norman Foster as a celebration of the age of air travel and as a symbol of the city's role as one of the world's great transport hubs, was deserted. Immigration and security officials outnumbered the handful of masked travellers still willing to travel on the empty flights to Hong Kong.

Those who could leave Hong Kong did so. Many of the city's expatriates sent their wives and children back to their home countries. Some decided that Hong Kong was not after all the land of opportunity they had thought it was and decided to leave for good. Wealthy locals with friends, relatives and homes overseas tried to leave as well. But many to their horror found they were not welcome abroad, but shunned as bearers of disease and forced to endure quarantines.

A city that had prided itself on being a place where the whole world came to make deals and do business now found itself shunned. Peripatetic business executives, who used Hong Kong as a base from which to make globe-girdling flights to serve markets and clients across the world, found themselves grounded as clients made it clear they did not want to see them just yet. The raw energy and drive that had transformed the barren island occupied by the British in 1841 into a gleaming hub of global commerce suddenly seemed to shrivel and dissipate under a cloud of uncertainty and fear. The Hang Seng Index of Hong Kong's blue chip stocks, the pulse of the city's business community, sputtered apologetically at levels that had not been seen since the Asian financial crisis in 1998.

Hong Kong had been through political and economic upheaval before. There had been the disruptions of the Cultural Revolution, when local radicals tried to emulate Mao's Red Guards. There had been the political uncertainty over Hong Kong's future during the long negotiations over the territory's return to Chinese sovereignty in 1997. There had been the Asian financial crisis. Hong Kong had ridden out each of these storms with the innate confidence of a city that has always lived and thrived by its wits.

But nothing had been this bad. Earlier crises had brought political and economic uncertainty. There had been the fear of losing deals, losing jobs and seeing fortunes shrink. But now, in addition to all of this, there was something new. There was the elemental fear of illness and death. And no one seemed to be exempt. It was not just those in crowded housing estates who were falling ill. The powerful and the wealthy were also at risk. One case of SARS had already been reported in the Peak, home to Hong Kong's wealthy. And a prominent public figure, William Ho, the head of the Hospital Authority, the body that runs Hong Kong's public hospital network, had fallen ill. In those dark days in March, SARS seemed to be a disease that could strike anyone, anytime.

Even so basic an activity as sending children to school seemed fraught with risk. Many parents followed their instincts and kept their children at home. Later the government would bow to public worries and shut schools and universities.

In this time of illness, even going to the doctor was a gamble. Who could be sure that the person sitting in the next seat in the doctor's waiting room was not ill with SARS? Even hospitals were no longer safe, with doctors and nurses, the frontline in the defence against disease, being hit the hardest. The disease seemed almost diabolical, laying bare a society's vulnerabilities by hitting at so many of the elements of normal life: sending children to school, going to the doctor or a hospital in the event of illness, taking a bus, visiting friends or being able to go to work without the fear of either spreading or catching a fatal infection.

* * *

It had been a Monday morning in late February when one of the early warnings of the disaster that lay ahead for Hong Kong first sounded. Andrew Yip, Chief of Surgery at Kwong Wah, a large, bustling hospital in the heart of the Kowloon district, was busy in his surgical ward on the seventh floor when he received a telephone call from Guangzhou.[1]

The caller at the other end was a Miss Tong, secretary to the Medical Superintendent of the Sun Yat Sen University of Medical Sciences. She had a favour to ask. An elderly professor of nephrology on their staff who was on a visit to Hong Kong had been admitted to Kwong Wah over the weekend and was understood to be in the Intensive Care Unit (ICU) with the respiratory disease that had been ravaging Guangdong province. "It is a very strange illness," the caller said. Could Yip arrange for a specialist to look at Professor Liu?

Yip went down two floors from his office in the surgery unit to the ICU to speak to its head, C L Watt.

Yes, they did have the professor from Guangdong, Liu Jianlun. He had come to the hospital two days ago on Saturday, February 23, feeling ill, and had warned hospital staff that he was probably suffering from the extremely contagious disease that he and his colleagues had been treating. "It is very dangerous," the professor had warned. The entire respiratory medicine team at his hospital in Guangzhou had fallen ill.

Liu told staff at Kwong Wah that he had first developed symptoms on February 15 and had treated himself with antibiotics. He had felt well enough to travel to Hong Kong for his nephew's wedding reception, but had begun to feel unwell the day he arrived in Hong Kong. After hearing his story, the staff at Kwong Wah decided to put the patient in isolation, and doctors and nurses wore masks before approaching him.

Later that day, there was another warning from Guangzhou. This time it came in the person of Zhan Wenhua, the Medical Superintendent of the Sun Yat Sen Medical College Hospital, where Professor Liu worked. Zhan had decided to travel to Hong Kong to check on his ailing colleague, and turned up at the Kwong Wah ICU on Monday evening. His message to the doctors in Hong Kong was as urgent as it was simple: please be very careful. The disease was extremely contagious. The entire respiratory medicine team at his hospital had come down with it. Even health workers who had not been in direct contact with patients had been infected. Please be very rigid on infection control, he urged.

Zhan said he and his colleagues in Guangzhou had no idea what was causing the disease. His hospital had found that treatment with steroids to reduce lung inflammation seemed to work. Before he left he had one question. "He asked us, 'Do you have any idea what is causing this?'" Andrew Yip recalled.

By this time, Liu's condition had deteriorated rapidly. He was heavily sedated, his lungs so full of fluid that he could not breathe without mechanical assistance. Yip was alarmed, and called up the best person he could think of, his good friend K Y Yuen, professor of microbiology at Hong Kong University. Yuen and Yip had been classmates at Hong Kong University Medical School, and Yip knew that if there was one person who knew about strange diseases, it was his old classmate.

K Y Yuen, a slim bespectacled man with a shock of floppy hair over his forehead that makes him look younger than his years, came over as soon as he could to look at the patient. He too was shocked by his first sight of a SARS patient. "Here was a man who had been perfectly healthy, now unconscious, struggling for his life in such a short time," he recalled. Yuen felt that this was a viral rather than a bacterial infection since the sick man had been treating himself with antibiotics, which would have cured a bacterial infection. Yuen advised that Liu Jianlun be treated with Ribavirin, an antiviral drug that was known to be active against a variety of viral agents.[2] Without the luxury of being able to conduct trials and studies on patients, Ribavirin would become the standard treatment for SARS in Hong Kong, though questions were later raised about how effective it was against the SARS virus.

Following Liu's arrival, there seemed little doubt among those who saw him in hospital that the mysterious disease that had been plaguing Guangdong was now in Hong Kong. For weeks Hong Kong had been hearing rumours about a disease raging across the border. Early in February, the press had carried reports of panic-stricken residents in Guangzhou raiding shops for medicines and masks to protect themselves. Then a sudden silence had fallen as the provincial authorities clamped down on media reporting of the disease and told the world that the epidemic had ended.

After the disease had broken out across the border, it was only a matter of time before it reached Hong Kong. Over 250 000 people cross the border between Hong Kong and the mainland every day, making it one of the busiest land crossings in the world. Viruses and diseases do not recognize or respect political boundaries, and any disease that is prevalent across the border will inevitably arrive in Hong Kong.

The health authorities in Hong Kong had in fact been on alert since early February for travellers bringing this new type of pneumonia into the territory. The Hospital Authority, the body that runs Hong Kong's public hospitals, had warned the hospitals under its management about the possibility of the disease crossing the border, and asked them to report any particularly severe cases of pneumonia in which the patient required oxygenation or intensive care.[3]

Hong Kong Health Department officials had tried to contact health officials in Guangdong to find out what was going on. But telephone calls to officials at the provincial health department as well as to Guangzhou city health officials were not returned. Faxed enquiries to these officials did not get any response either.[4] The lack of response was not unusual. Though Hong Kong and Guangdong are neighbouring regions of China, Hong Kong has very little official contact with its neighbour. As part of the political arrangements that accompanied the return of Hong Kong to Chinese sovereignty after more than 150 years of British colonial rule, the territory has a special autonomous status within China. As a result, it has little to do with neighbouring provinces, and deals directly with the Central government in Beijing. At the time these arrangements were made, it was thought that insulating Hong Kong in this way would help preserve its autonomy. But as SARS demonstrated, this lack of communication and coordination between adjoining regions is dysfunctional.

In the absence of concrete information about the situation in Guangdong, the Hospital Authority sent out a general warning about severe cases of pneumonia. Because of this warning, when Professor Liu turned up at Kwong Wah Hospital, his case was reported up the chain of command to the Hospital Authority and the Department of Health.

But the Department of Health did not act on this information with the seriousness that it required. This would be one of the policy errors in the battle against SARS; that despite being on the alert for a contagious disease from Guangdong, when a case actually turned up, nothing was done to inform medical workers or the general public. It was only two weeks later, after an outbreak among doctors and nurses at the Prince of Wales Hospital, that it would be acknowledged that Hong Kong was in the grip of an epidemic. After Professor Liu's admission and subsequent death, why was nothing done about the fact that a contagious disease of unknown origins was on the loose?

The Department of Health continues to react defensively to suggestions that it missed a major opportunity to alert Hong Kong and the rest of the world to the presence of a new contagious disease. But an investigation of the department's actions after it was informed about the case at Kwong Wah Hospital shows that its response was overly bureaucratic. There appears to have been a lack of suspicion about the arrival of an unusual case of pneumonia from Guangzhou.

When it was informed on February 24 of the presence of a severe case of pneumonia from Guangzhou in Hong Kong, the Health Department, in accordance with its normal procedures, sent a nurse to Kwong Wah Hospital to interview the patient. Liu, sedated and intubated, was in no condition to be interviewed. So the nurse copied his case notes, and then rang his wife, sister and daughter to see whether they were well. Liu's brother-in-law and wife were unwell, and so the nurse urged them to go to the nearest hospital. His wife decided to return to Guangzhou, where she was diagnosed with SARS but later recovered.[5]

Liu's brother-in-law was admitted to Kwong Wah Hospital and later died of SARS. Two nurses at the hospital fell ill as well. This was the same pattern that had been seen in Guangzhou: a highly infectious disease spreading among hospital workers and close contacts of patients. But these new infections did not trigger any alarm, and no wider alert was sent out by the Department of Health.

When legislators in Hong Kong questioned the government about this, they received a disingenuous response from the then Director of

Health, Margaret Chan. "No one suspected the disease from which Professor Liu died was contagious."[6] This assertion flew in the face of facts. The Department of Health must have known the disease was contagious: two family members of the patient and two health care workers had already fallen ill.

Several factors appear to have contributed to the Department of Health's response. The first was the misinformation coming from the Guangdong provincial government about the magnitude of the outbreak there. As discussed earlier, on February 11, the Guangdong provincial authorities announced that the epidemic was under control, after infecting 305 people between December 2002 and early February 2003. The Hong Kong health authorities as well as the WHO initially took this statement at face value. Three hundred five cases of pneumonia in a province of 50 million people was not a major health scare. Because of the small numbers, and the assurances that the epidemic had died out, the Hong Kong health authorities did not see the arrival of the disease in Hong Kong as a major public health risk. Also, the disease had been described in China as an "atypical pneumonia," a term that would cover any pneumonia caused by an agent other than common microbes such as the *streptococcus* bacteria. Atypical pneumonias are not a cause for alarm, and the presence of an atypical pneumonia in Guangdong did not ring any major warnings.

The second factor was that Hong Kong's public health system was very narrowly focused on the threat of a possible influenza epidemic. A week before Professor Liu's admission to hospital, Hong Kong had its first two human cases of H5N1 influenza since 1997. H5N1 influenza is normally confined to birds, but when it does cross over to humans, it is lethal. In 1997, six of the 18 people who caught the disease died and the Hong Kong government ordered the slaughter of the territory's chicken population to stop the disease from spreading. With new cases of H5N1 emerging at the same time as reports of a mysterious new disease in China, the Department of Health was primarily interested in trying to determine whether the disease in Guangdong was bird flu, and whether Professor Liu was suffering from bird flu. When tests showed that Liu was not suffering from influenza, his illness was regarded as just another unusual form of pneumonia, and nothing more was thought of it.

There was also a reluctance to examine anecdotal evidence coming from southern China about the severity of the disease and its infectiousness.[7] Had this been done, and had a general alert been sent to hospitals and doctors to be extremely suspicious about all cases of pneumonia and to adopt the strictest infection control measures, SARS might not have spread the way it did in Hong Kong.

Indeed, SARS might not have flared up into a major global epidemic except for a chain of unusual circumstances, some of which are still not fully understood. Professor Liu was not the first patient with SARS in Hong Kong. There were at least two earlier cases. On January 22, before SARS was recognized as a new disease, a patient who had travelled to mainland China was admitted to the Pamela Youde Nethersole Hospital in Hong Kong with severe pneumonia, and died on February 3.[8] The disease did not spread in the hospital, and the case was recorded as another case of pneumonia. Months later, stored serum samples from the patient tested positive for SARS, indicating that at least one case of SARS had arrived in Hong Kong by as early as the end of January.

On February 17, five days before Professor Liu turned up at hospital, a 49-year-old Hong Kong woman had fallen ill while visiting her mother in Henan, in Guangdong province. She returned to Hong Kong with symptoms of pneumonia and admitted herself to Union Hospital, a private hospital in the New Territories. She became worse, and was transferred to the ICU of the larger Prince of Wales Hospital, where she recovered and was discharged. Once again, the disease did not spread into the community from this early case, although one nurse who had treated her at Union Hospital fell ill a few days later, recovering after five days in hospital. Later, her blood serum samples showed she had also contracted SARS.

It was Professor Liu who triggered the epidemic in Hong Kong and globally. All of Vietnam's 63 SARS cases, as well as 238 cases in Singapore and 136 cases in Canada flowed directly or indirectly from this one person. A fateful chain of events, first in a dim hotel corridor, then in a busy hospital ward and finally in a nondescript apartment complex would magnify and transform the virus-laden exhalations of an elderly man into a global public health emergency.

* * *

By the time Professor Liu was admitted to Kwong Wah Hospital, the SARS virus had already begun its journey around the world. Either on the night of February 22 or the morning of February 23, in the unlikely surroundings of the Metropole Hotel, a well-run, pleasant, mid-range hotel popular with package tourists, an unknown event would take place that would allow the SARS virus to jump from the elderly doctor to a group of people who would then transport it across the world.

Liu and his wife checked into the Metropole on Friday evening, February 22. The elderly couple had come to Hong Kong to celebrate the wedding of Liu's nephew and had arrived earlier in the day from Guangzhou. They had spent most of the day with Liu's sister, brother-in-law and other family members. When they checked into the hotel that night after a family dinner, Liu was already tired. He spent a restless night, feeling increasingly feverish. The next day, his son and daughter arrived from Guangzhou, but Liu felt so ill that he went to the nearest hospital, Kwong Wah, barely a mile down the road from the Metropole Hotel.

During that brief period between the late evening of February 22 and the morning of February 23, something happened in the passageway between Liu's room, number 911, and the lifts located about 20 metres away that allowed the SARS virus to make the fatal jump that would lead to a global health emergency.

Fate had brought together a disparate group of people on the ninth floor of the Metropole Hotel on those two days. A few doors away from Professor Liu and his wife were another elderly couple who had come to Hong Kong on a family visit. Kwan Suichu, a 78-year-old grandmother from Toronto and her husband had come to visit their sons over the Chinese New Year. They had spent most of their two weeks in Hong Kong with their sons, but were spending Friday, February 22, the last night of their stay, at the Metropole Hotel as part of an airline-hotel package deal.

Staying in the room opposite to Liu's was Johnny Cheng, the Shanghai-based manager of a New York textile company. Cheng would leave for Vietnam two days later on February 25 to visit his company's garment factory in Hanoi.

At one end of the corridor was 23-year-old Esther Mok, a former airline stewardess from Singapore who was with a friend on a shopping trip. In a nearby room was the guide from their tour group. Also on the same corridor was a 72-year-old Chinese-Canadian of Hong Kong origin who was back to catch up with friends and family over the Chinese New Year.

No one knows when, or even if, this group of people met in the hotel, and how they got the virus from Professor Liu. None of those who are still alive recall seeing him on the evening of the 21st or the morning of the 22nd. Months later, epidemiologists were still baffled by how the elderly professor, who spent most of his time in his room after checking in, could have spread the virus to this group of people. Investigators subjected the hotel rooms of each of the patients to minute

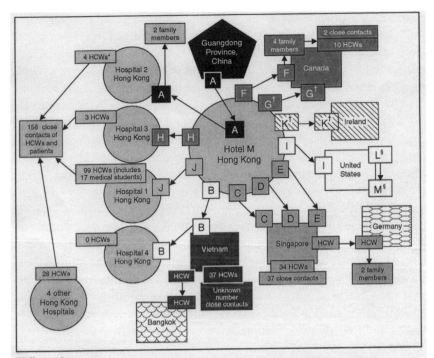

*Health-care workers.
†All guests except G and K stayed on the 9th floor of the hotel. Guest G stayed on the 14th floor, and Guest K stayed on the 11th floor.
§Guests L and M (spouses) were not at Hotel M during the same time as index Guest A but were at the hotel during the same times as Guests G, H, and I, who were ill during this period.

How SARS spread from the Metropole Hotel (courtesy: Centers for Disease Control and Prevention, Atlanta, Morbidity and Mortality Weekly Report).

examination, taking samples from carpets, furniture, air vents and toilets for examination. The samples revealed no trace of the virus. Whatever happened occurred outside the rooms.

Most of those who were infected at the hotel had rooms on the same wing as Professor Liu. This indicates that the virus was transmitted in the common corridor in front of their rooms rather than in the hotel's main lobby or any of the other public areas. Had the virus been passed on in a more public place, this would have infected people in a large number of rooms, rather than those on a single wing of one floor.

Molecular examination of the carpeting in the hallway in front of Liu's room, as well as the lift area a few feet away, revealed tiny slivers of genetic material from the SARS virus, the only traces of the virus found anywhere in the hotel. "There was a contamination of some sort in the hallway," Heinz Feldmann, the head of a WHO investigative team would later report. "Maybe the professor vomited in the evening and it was cleaned up either by himself or his wife."[9] But Liu's wife, whom Hong Kong Department of Health officials contacted in China, could not remember him vomiting or spitting in the hallway. The Metropole Hotel staff too could not remember cleaning up anything in the hallway.

"We have circumstantial evidence that something happened in the hallway, but the missing link is the actual history of what happened," explained Thomas Tsang, the Hong Kong Department of Health epidemiologist who was involved in the investigation. "The professor has passed away, his wife cannot recall any such incident, and there were no surveillance cameras that recorded anything. So we don't know."[10]

Equally mysterious is the fact that one person who was not on the ninth floor, a 55-year-old Vancouver man who was staying on the 16th floor of the hotel, was infected. He would later become the index patient for the SARS outbreak in British Columbia. Also infected was a 26-year-old Hong Kong man who was not even a guest at the hotel, but had merely visited a friend on the ninth floor. It was this man who would unwittingly cause the major outbreak of the disease at the Prince of Wales Hospital in Hong Kong.

How the virus was passed on remains a mystery. All that is known is that it was passed on extremely efficiently. Like human bombs, these initial victims would in turn set off explosive chains of infection that could all be traced back to a fleeting encounter in an anonymous hallway in an unremarkable Hong Kong hotel.

In the aftermath of any catastrophic event, it is always tempting to second guess history, and this is true in the case of SARS. Had that group of people not stayed at the Metropole Hotel, would the course of history have been different? Would the world have been spared an epidemic that crippled so many cities and cost so many lives?

The answer is no. The definitive moment in the SARS epidemic was when the new virus first emerged in the human population some time in late 2002. Once it had begun spreading in the human population in southern China, and given the relative ease with which it spread, it was only a matter of time before it spread to the wider world. The only way a global epidemic could have been prevented was if the disease had been contained in southern China. Once it was allowed to spread in Guangdong province, it would inevitably cross to Hong Kong and from there to the wider world.

Had that group of people not been at the Metropole Hotel, their individual histories, and the histories of those whom they infected, would have been different. Many of those who are dead today would still be alive. But the disease itself would have spread, although through other people and under different circumstances. Instead of an elderly doctor in a hotel corridor infecting other guests, it might well have been some other traveller from southern China infecting a group of people in another setting — in an airport perhaps, or on a plane.

Many of those from this small group at the Metropole were later identified as the "index cases" who brought the disease from Hong Kong to their home countries, and were unfairly stigmatized for a blind accident of fate. Disease, like nature, strikes blindly. All human beings can do is to take precautions if they are forewarned. In the case of SARS, ordinary people had no forewarning and there were no precautions they could take. The travellers at the Metropole Hotel had blundered unknowingly into what was to be the greatest tragedy of their lives.

▲ ▲ ▲

In Hong Kong, those who had been infected at the Metropole Hotel by Professor Liu took the disease to four public hospitals. But it was from only one of these hospitals, the Prince of Wales Hospital, that the epidemic spread to the wider community.

The first hospital to receive SARS patients was the Kwong Wah Hospital, where Professor Liu and his brother-in-law infected two hospital workers. Staff members were aware that Liu's disease was dangerous and contagious, and had taken infection control precautions, so the spread in the hospital was limited.

The second cluster of infection was started by another of the guests on the ninth floor of the Metropole, the 72-year-old Canadian-Chinese man who was on holiday in Hong Kong. He had been staying at the hotel since the middle of February, but there was just one night, February 21, when he and Liu could have crossed paths. Like the other ill-fated hotel guests, he started feeling feverish the following week, and after seeing a doctor, admitted himself on March 2 to St Paul's, a small Catholic hospital in Hong Kong's Causeway Bay district. Here, he infected three nurses and a fellow patient two beds away from him who was recovering from a kidney ailment. His 50-year-old nephew, who had visited him at the Metropole Hotel and at St. Paul's, also caught SARS.

Four days later, as his condition worsened, the elderly Canadian was transferred to Queen Mary Hospital, the teaching hospital of the Hong Kong University Medical School. Here, he was treated for pneumonia, initially in a general ward, and later in the hospital's ICU.

His nephew and the kidney patient he had infected at St Paul's would also be admitted to Queen Mary. But at Queen Mary the disease was contained, and did not spread among the hospital staff (except for two cases a month later) or out into the community.

The epidemic in Hong Kong erupted at the Prince of Wales Hospital, one of Hong Kong's largest and best equipped hospitals.[11] It is the teaching hospital for the Chinese University of Hong Kong, one of the territory's two top universities. It was to this busy, sprawling hospital in the New Territories town of Shatin that a 26-year-old local man who has only been identified as "Mr C" went on February 28, complaining that he had been suffering from high fever and body aches for the past three days. Mr C had been infected when he visited a friend on the ninth floor of the Metropole Hotel. He was seen at the hospital's emergency department, and sent home with medication.

The man reappeared on March 4 feeling breathless and displaying symptoms of pneumonia. He was ill enough to be admitted to hospital, and was given a bed in Ward 8A, one of the hospital's medical wards. Within weeks, this otherwise ordinary hospital ward would be known around the world as the site of Hong Kong's SARS explosion.

Ward 8A is reserved for male patients, and looks like any other busy public hospital ward in a developed country anywhere in the world. Its 30 beds are usually filled with patients of every age, shape and size displaying a rich variety of ailments. Since no one in Hong Kong was aware of SARS as a disease, Mr C was thought to be just another case of community-acquired pneumonia, a condition that is not uncommon in Hong Kong at that time of year. The only slightly unusual element was that he was in his twenties, while pneumonia tends to affect older patients with weaker immune systems.

Mr C was treated with antibiotics, and after a week in hospital, his fever diminished and the patches on his lungs started to disappear. But during those first few days in hospital, he coughed and coughed. His airways were choked with phlegm and he found it almost impossible to breathe. So the doctors ordered a procedure that is common in such cases, but will probably never be used again at the Prince of Wales Hospital. They used a nebulizer — a device that delivers drugs to the lungs and respiratory passages in the form of a fine mist — to clear his airways.

A nebulizer is an excellent way to deliver drugs to patients with respiratory difficulties. But it is also a supremely efficient way for any viruses or bacteria within the respiratory tract to reach the outside world. Each inhalation, during which the drug is pushed into the lungs, is followed by an exhalation, when air, as well as any infectious particles, is pushed out of the lungs and respiratory tract into the outside world. At the time Mr C was being nebulized, his upper respiratory tract would have been swarming with rapidly multiplying colonies of hundreds of millions of SARS coronaviruses. Each nebulized exhalation was like an expressway for the virus to the larger world. The nebulizer also aerosolized the patient's virus-laden exhalations, allowing the virus to travel much further than the one metre a droplet normally travels.

Mr C was given a drug to dilate his bronchial passage through a nebulizer four times a day for seven days. On each of those 28 occasions, every breath he exhaled contained an invisible mist of millions of viral particles that would drift in a deadly cloud above the beds and passageways of the busy ward, lingering in the air and settling at random on other patients, nurses, doctors, medical equipment, tables, chairs and beds.

Four medical teams — one team of doctors and three teams of nurses — minister to the needs of the 30-odd patients in Ward 8A. A few days after Mr C's arrival on March 4, a few team members began to feel feverish and unwell. By the beginning of the second week of March, third year medical students who had been brought to Ward 8A by their professors to examine patients and demonstrate their clinical skills were also beginning to feel unwell.

Henry Chan, a youthful-looking associate professor of medicine at Chinese University, had brought three of his students to Ward 8A on March 7 to test their skills in examining patients and diagnosing illness. When he has students to test, Chan normally chooses patients who are relatively well and cheerful enough to put up with the often fumbling questions and probing of would-be doctors. So he avoided Mr C, who seemed far too sick to be a useful guinea pig, and pointed his students towards other, more amenable patients. As Chan recalled, he did not go close to Mr C, or even spend long in the ward. But the amount of virus in the air and on the surfaces of the hospital ward was enough to infect him.[12]

Three mornings later, on March 10, he woke with a fever and headache, and thinking he had the flu, called in sick and tried to sleep off the illness. What he did not know was that 50 of his fellow doctors, nurses and nursing assistants, all of whom worked on the eighth floor medical wards, had also fallen sick.

His boss, Joseph Sung, the hospital's chief physician, was extremely worried. Sung had been travelling abroad and arrived back the previous day to the news that 12 of his staff had fallen sick. By the next day, this number had jumped alarmingly. Though doctors and nurses are in contact with sick patients every day, when they all fall ill at the same time, it is a clear indication that something is seriously wrong.

Sung, like everyone else in the medical profession in Hong Kong, was aware that there had been an outbreak of pneumonia across the border in Guangdong, but had few details about the disease. He had no idea that the disease had arrived in Hong Kong, and that Kwong Wah Hospital already had four cases: Professor Liu, his brother-in-law and two nurses.[13]

Sung, however, did call a fellow professor he knew at the Sun Yat Sen Medical University in Guangzhou to ask him about the disease. He got the same message that every doctor who had dealt with SARS would repeat: this was a very serious illness, it was extremely contagious and many health care workers had been infected. Doctors and nurses treating patients had to take every precaution; medical workers in Guangdong had started changing clothes and protective gear and showering several times a day.

Fearing that he could be facing an extremely serious outbreak of pneumonia, Sung decided to ask all of the doctors, nurses and health assistants who had called in sick to come into the hospital for a check-up. Given the warnings about how infectious the disease was, he wanted to keep any infected staff members in isolation so they did not spread the disease. An observation ward in the Prince of Wales emergency department with its own air-conditioning system and a separate entrance was requisitioned for use as a makeshift ward for afflicted hospital workers.

When Henry Chan came in for his check-up, he found the room full of sick doctors and nurses. "The corridor was full of my colleagues," he recalled.[14] Each of them was X-rayed, and temperatures were taken. All of them had fever, and many were showing signs of pneumonia. Twenty-three of the worst affected, including Chan, found themselves admitted to an isolation ward.

"We checked 50 health care workers that night. All of them had signs of fever and pneumonia. We did not have space to admit all of them, so I only took in 23 of the most serious cases. If we had space for all of them, I would have admitted all 50," Sung recalled.[15]

Chan was not particularly worried at first. Like any group of sick doctors, he and his colleagues quickly dissected their symptoms and concluded that whatever the cause of their illness, it was viral. "I knew it was viral," Chan recalled. "My white blood cell count indicated it was viral, and with a bacterial infection, it would also be easier to locate the place of infection. With this illness, there just seemed to be general fever, aches and pains." He concluded this was a flu virus with slightly unusual symptoms.

The next day, Chan woke up to find his fever gone. "I felt better, so I discharged myself and went home." A day later he would be back in hospital though, with the high fever, aches and breathing difficulty typical of SARS. This time he spent two and a half weeks in hospital, much of it racked with fever and the worst cough he had ever experienced. "I coughed so badly, I couldn't talk. And I was so weak that I could hardly go to the toilet on my own. And I had constant chills and muscle pains."

Those first few weeks in March at the Prince of Wales Hospital were a hospital administrator's worst nightmare come to life. This new plague kept spreading relentlessly, first striking doctors, nurses, hospital workers and other patients, and then spreading out of the hospital into the community as the families of doctors and health care workers and the friends and relatives of patients fell ill. Through the second week of March, the numbers rose steadily by ones and twos every day as the staff and patients of Ward 8A succumbed. Then their family members, friends and relatives began to fall ill, indicating that the disease was establishing itself in the wider community. It was clear that the hospital, in a cruel reversal of its normal role, was acting as an amplifier for the disease, spreading it both within the hospital and out into the community.

For doctors and other hospital personnel, whether healthy or ill, it was perhaps the most traumatic period in their careers. For those who fell ill, the pain, discomfort and fear of confronting a new disease somehow seemed harder when colleagues were ill alongside them, and other colleagues were treating them.

"It was perhaps a mistake putting all of them together," said Joseph Sung. "Many of them got worse at first, and they could see each other falling more and more ill, and they could all see and compare each other's charts. They just got more and more worried."[16] The infected medical workers were in a windowless ward, with little to distract them. Those who were well enough watched television. What they saw on the news made them even more worried. As the epidemic spread through Hong Kong, the streets were emptying, people were wearing masks, and a cloud of fear had settled over the city.

Those who stayed well and had to run the hospital faced one of the hardest professional challenges of their lives. "This was a terrible time for me," Sung recalled. "I had a crisis on my hands. I had a lot of young colleagues who looked up to me, and expected me to provide them with answers. Many of them were getting worse, and being transferred to the Intensive Care Unit. So I tried to keep a cheerful appearance, talk to all of them. I couldn't look helpless, so I put on a strong face and tried to cheer them all up."

As SARS spread through Ward 8A and out into the wider community, questions would be asked about why the infection had been able to spread in this way. SARS is a virus spread through droplets. Why were basic infection control measures against droplet infection not carried out, and if they were, why had they failed?

Some of the strongest questioning came from Hong Kong University and Queen Mary Hospital. Doctors at Queen Mary pointed out that the Prince of Wales and Queen Mary each admitted one patient from the initial group of cases infected at the Metropole Hotel. At that time, neither hospital knew that these were SARS patients. Yet the disease only spread from the Prince of Wales Hospital and not Queen Mary. Administrators at Queen Mary pointed out that only two nurses contracted SARS at Queen Mary, compared to the 160 nurses, doctors and assistants infected at the Prince of Wales. Doctors at Queen Mary attributed the difference to the tighter infection control measures implemented at Queen Mary.

"We are the infection control hospital in Hong Kong," Dr Seto Wing Hong, the head of infection control at Queen Mary, explained. "Infection control is not something you can do overnight. This is something we have been drilling into staff for years. We have inculcated this culture, and it paid off."[17]

To the doctors at Queen Mary and the medical faculty at Hong Kong University, it would appear to be negligence at the Prince of Wales that had allowed the epidemic to spread from a hospital ward to the rest of the community. In a letter to the newspapers, the Dean of the Hong Kong University Medical School, Lam Shiu-kum, noted:

> The real outbreak was a hospital outbreak, which occurred in the Prince of Wales Hospital. The majority of cases in Hong Kong originated from one ward where one index patient was treated. The virus spread to the doctors, nurses, medical students, other health workers and visitors...The most disturbing aspect, however, is that the index patient with atypical pneumonia was admitted to the Prince of Wales after the outbreak in Guangzhou had been in the news, and after it had been reported that a patient with atypical pneumonia had been admitted to Kwong Wah Hospital.[18]

Doctors at the Prince of Wales were outraged. In an open letter, 100 doctors from the hospital claimed that these charges had damaged the morale of frontline staff at the hospital, who had "been labouring under extreme stress for more than four weeks." The Prince of Wales doctors also argued that Queen Mary had been better prepared because it had known about Professor Liu's hospitalization at Kwong Wah Hospital before the Prince of Wales.[19]

It didn't help that after the initial round of infections at the Prince of Wales, Ward 8A was involved in two other outbreaks, including one that resulted in the spread of the disease to the Chinese province of Inner Mongolia. On March 15, a 72-year-old man who had become infected with SARS while visiting a relative in Ward 8A boarded a flight from Hong Kong to Beijing. In the course of the three-hour flight, he infected 21 other passengers and crew members, some sitting as far as seven seats away from him. The two stewardesses on the flight were both from Inner Mongolia, and both took SARS back to their homes, setting off a chain of nearly 300 infections in the province.

It was also as a result of the infection in Ward 8A that SARS broke out in the Amoy Gardens housing complex. In Hong Kong's campaign against SARS, Amoy Gardens was the defining battle. Had it been lost, the numbers of SARS cases could have multiplied so rapidly that the territory's health care system would have collapsed.

* * *

It started with a 33-year-old man from Shenzhen, the mainland boom town just across the border from Hong Kong. He was being treated on a long-term basis for a kidney ailment at the Prince of Wales Hospital, and had a brother who lived at Amoy Gardens and whom he visited frequently. On March 15, the kidney patient had turned up at the Prince of Wales with symptoms of SARS, and was admitted to Ward 8A. The previous day, he had stayed with his brother at Amoy Gardens. The man was diagnosed with influenza, and discharged from hospital on March 19, after he seemed to have recovered. Once again, he stayed with his brother and sister-in-law at Amoy Gardens. His symptoms reappeared over the next few days, and on March 22 he went back to the Prince of Wales, where he was readmitted.

Meanwhile, his brother and sister-in-law at Amoy Gardens were starting to feel unwell. Doctors in the area began noticing an unusual number of patients turning up with fevers and pneumonia-like symptoms. It was on March 25 that Osmond Kwok, a doctor with a clinic a stone's throw away from Amoy Gardens, began noticing an unusual number of patients turning up with fever and pneumonia symptoms.[20] Kwok would normally expect to see one or two patients with pneumonia in a month. But now he was suddenly getting two and three a day. He followed the government's recommendation to treat patients with antibiotics for two days and then send them for chest X-rays if they showed no improvement. By March 27, he realized that the majority of his patients were not getting better, and were developing tell-tale patches on their lungs. Within the next few days, he would see 20 patients with SARS-like symptoms, 14 of whom would later be confirmed to have the disease. Like other doctors working in the area, Kwok was concerned and uncertain about what to do. "What really worried me was the thought that doctors all over Hong Kong might be seeing the same number of cases. I thought this might be part of a huge outbreak all over Hong Kong. I couldn't know at the time that this was only in Amoy Gardens."[21] But what Kwok was seeing in his clinic was causing alarm elsewhere.

Queen's Road East is a typically busy Hong Kong thoroughfare, cluttered with traffic and lined with every conceivable kind of building from high-rise office towers to dilapidated apartment buildings. It is here, on the 18th floor of an office complex that houses the Department of Health's communicable disease unit, that Thomas Tsang, the department's top epidemiologist, works. A slightly built, energetic man, Tsang had been working 18-hour days since the beginning of March, gathering data to monitor the spread of the disease and setting up systems to track the people with whom SARS patients had been in contact and who they might have passed the disease on to.

On March 26, he noticed that the United Christian Hospital, the public hospital that serves the Amoy Gardens area, had reported 15 SARS cases in a single day, all with addresses from Amoy Gardens. "That's very alarming, to get 15 cases from a single address, so we immediately went there to take a look," Tsang said. "Our first thought was that perhaps they had met at a common gathering, perhaps gone to a restaurant together or a church or gone on a tour together."[22] But there was no such link.

While the Department of Health tried to determine the cause of the outbreak, the numbers of cases from the building complex were leaping at a rate that had not been seen in Hong Kong or anywhere else in the world so far. On March 27, 27 people from Amoy Gardens were hospitalized. The next day, 34 more were admitted to hospital. The day after that it was 36. On March 31, 64 more people were taken to hospital. By now the bulk of new cases in Hong Kong were from this

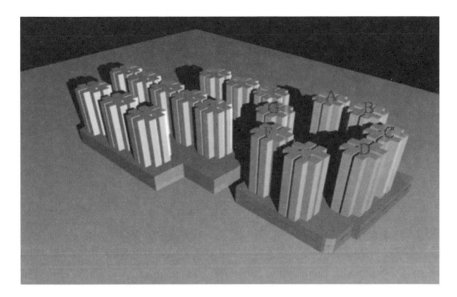

Plan of Amoy Gardens (courtesy: Stephen Ng)

one housing complex. And within the housing complex, most cases were from Block E.

Between March 26 and March 31, the complexion of the threat that Hong Kong faced from SARS seemed to change. Until then, public health officials were reasonably certain that this disease was transmitted through droplets from infected people, and that the only way for fresh infections to occur was through contact with people who were already ill. The strategy for controlling an epidemic being transmitted in this way is reasonably simple: tighten infection control in hospitals and introduce tracing of people who come in contact with known cases.

But the Amoy Gardens outbreak could not be explained through droplet transmission alone. The virus was spreading in a new, unknown way, and it was spreading much faster. It had apparently found some way of transmitting through the environment. What was this new method of transmission? Equally important, would this new method appear all over Hong Kong, or was it due to an unusual set of circumstances that would not be replicated?

The answers to these questions had implications not only for Hong Kong, but globally as well. If the SARS virus had in fact found a second method of transmission, then the global strategy to control the epidemic would have to be re-examined. The strategy that the WHO had developed was based on the belief that SARS spread through droplets, and that its transmission could be stopped by identifying those at risk and isolating them in hospital. If this disease could spread through the environment, this strategy would be useless.

For Hong Kong, the ability of the health system to cope with the disease was at stake. As the number of cases sky-rocketed in the last week of March due to the Amoy Gardens outbreak, there was a danger that the hospital system would collapse. The system was already beginning to buckle under the twin pressures of increasing numbers of SARS patients and a decreasing number of doctors and nurses available to provide care.

By the last week of March, the numbers of new cases coming in had reached 100 a day. In the first three weeks of the SARS outbreak, 524 cases had been reported. But if 100 new patients started coming in every day, this figure would double in just five days. Hong Kong's public hospital system had the capacity to handle 3000 cases of SARS. Unless the rate at which the epidemic was growing slowed, by the end of April, the system would no longer be able to cope.

The crisis was most acute in the ICUs, which were filling up with SARS patients. Hong Kong's public hospitals have 400 ICU beds. By the end of March, 150 of them had been filled. If the number of new cases continued to increase, and if the number of SARS patients needing intensive care remained at the current rate of around 25 percent, then the system would break down.

The key to avoiding this impending disaster was to stop the spread at Amoy Gardens, and to understand what it was that was causing this explosion in the housing complex. Once that was understood, it would be possible to determine whether this was an unusual occurrence or a method of transmission that could become common across Hong Kong.

The first step was to prevent Amoy Gardens residents from spreading the disease outside the complex. The only way to do this was to impose a quarantine on the building. Hong Kong had been toying with the idea of invoking mandatory quarantine regulations in the same way that Singapore had done. But it had hesitated to do so. In Singapore it was possible for the government to back up its diktat with swift punishment. In Hong Kong this was not possible. But as the Amoy Gardens outbreak exploded, the government decided it had no option but to use its powers to prevent people from spreading the disease further. On March 27, Chief Executive Tung Chee-hwa announced that the Quarantine and Prevention of Disease Ordinance would be invoked to ensure that those who had been in close contact with SARS patients did not wander around at will.

On March 31, as the number of cases from Amoy Gardens continued to rise, the government clamped an isolation order on Block E, preventing anyone from leaving or entering the building. The next day, residents were bussed out and an army of investigators got to work, subjecting every inch of the 20-year-old building to minute examination in the search for clues as to how the virus was spreading through it.

Block E of Amoy Gardens was built in 1981, and its utilitarian design and architecture are typical of many middle-income housing developments built in Hong Kong during this period. Each floor of the cruciform-shaped building has eight apartments, each approximately 48 square metres in area. There were a few clues as to how SARS might have spread in the building. The first was that the majority of those who had fallen ill lived in two vertical lines of flats: flats 7 and 8 of each floor. Flat 8 on every floor seemed to be the hardest hit, with residents in 73 percent of these units reporting infection. Also, while there were cases from other blocks, those who lived in Block E had fallen ill about three days earlier, indicating that this block was where the infection had first broken out.

The investigators collected every possible kind of sample — from the air, the water and the sewage system, as well as from cockroaches, rats, cats and dogs in and around the building. "At first we looked at the water tanks a lot and thought it might be contaminated water that was spreading the virus," explained Thomas Tsang, the Health Department epidemiologist. But the water samples were clean. "We thought it might be something in the garbage, but there was nothing once again to show that there was a source of virus in the garbage that was passing into apartments."[23]

The vertical pattern in which the flats had been infected was clearly a clue, but a clue to what? "At one moment we thought it might be a biological attack because of the vertical arrangement of cases," said Tsang. This possibility was quickly dismissed

The air and water proved to be clean. Traces of the coronavirus were found in the bodies of cockroaches and in rat droppings. But cockroaches would not account for the unique distribution of the infected flats. If cockroaches were to blame, they would have carried the virus horizontally among all the flats on a single floor, and not only vertically, as was the case in Amoy Gardens. Also, while rodent droppings contained the virus, the rats themselves did not carry it. The rats could possibly have acted as carriers, but the Health Department epidemiologists felt this would not account for the pattern in which apartments in the building were being infected.

It was around this time that researchers found that the SARS coronavirus was also excreted in the faeces of infected people, and that it could survive in this medium for some time. The only trace of virus found in any of the apartments was on the toilet rim of one apartment. It was also known that unusually, most of the patients from Amoy Gardens had diarrhoea in addition to the common SARS symptoms. The patient from the Prince of Wales Hospital who had triggered the outbreak had been suffering from diarrhoea and was known to have used the toilet several times during his stay. Had this been the source of infection, and had the virus leaked in some way from the sewage system and infected residents all over the building?

The question was how. "If you think there is virus in the faeces in the sewer pipe that has caused all these infections, then you have to find out how it got from the sewage pipes into the flat," explained Tsang. Given the construction of the bathrooms in the apartments, there were two ways that sewage could flow back in: through the toilets, and through the bathroom floor drains, which are connected to the sewage pipes.

Examination of the floor drains revealed that the U-traps, bends in the pipe that are meant to prevent a reflux of sewage, were dry. In order to function, these traps must be filled with water. Those who had designed the apartments had assumed that people would wash their bathroom floors with water every day, and that this water would flow down into the floor drains and fill the traps. In the early 1980s, when the apartments were built, this was a common practice. But over time, people had begun adopting a more modern and convenient way of cleaning their floors by mopping them. This meant that the floor drains fell into disuse, and the water in the U-traps dried out.

Even with the traps dry, sewage would not automatically flow back into the bathrooms. This would require some mechanism that created negative air pressure in the bathrooms, sucking sewage droplets back into the bathrooms. As they examined every feature of the tiny bathrooms, the investigators focused on the exhaust fans fitted into the top of the bathroom windows. These fans had not been part of the original design but had been added by flat owners in order to ventilate the bathrooms. If the exhaust fan was on, and the bathroom door shut, would enough negative pressure be created to pull droplets in from the waste pipes?

Tsang and his investigators decided to find out. They stuck strips of paper over the grill on bathroom drains, shut the doors and turned on the exhaust fans. The paper strips lifted up in the powerful air current that was formed, clearly indicating that air was being sucked in from the drain pipes. If the exhaust fans were on when people used the shower, sewage droplets and the moisture from the shower could mix and settle on bathroom surfaces. This experiment showed that it was theoretically possible for droplets of sewage to be sucked into the bathrooms and infect people. But was this what really happened? To test their theory, Tsang had his colleagues set up a classic epidemiological study, interviewing residents about their behaviour and comparing the rates of infection among those who used the exhaust fans with those who did not. The results showed that those who had used their exhaust fans while taking a shower had a five times greater chance of getting SARS than those who did not use the fan, indicating that this was probably how the contamination occurred.

There was another factor that could have allowed the virus to pass from the bathroom in one flat to bathrooms in other flats on higher floors. All the apartments in Amoy Gardens are connected through a light well — an enclosed space that contains the plumbing and water pipes from each unit, and which also acts as a ventilation source for the bathrooms. Experiments conducted by a WHO team showed that the pressure generated by the exhaust fans was strong enough to draw contaminated droplets from bathrooms into the light well, from where droplets could have entered other flats through the bathroom windows.

The conclusion of the Health Department was that the infection at Amoy Gardens had been started by the kidney patient, who had initially infected a small number of people through direct contact during his stay at the housing complex. These people had fallen ill, and begun shedding the virus into the sewage system, from where it had entered other apartments through the floor drains and been deposited on bathroom surfaces and toiletries.

These findings were good news for Hong Kong. If dried-out floor drains were the main cause of the outbreak, then it was easy to prevent future contamination by ensuring that the U-traps remained filled with water. If viral particles were also transmitted through light wells, then keeping bathroom windows closed would be a simple preventive measure. Most importantly, the findings indicated that the Amoy Gardens outbreak was the result of an unusual set of circumstances rather than a forewarning of similar outbreaks in housing complexes throughout Hong Kong. As a WHO investigative team put it, "It seems highly likely that an unfortunate sequence of environmental and health events happened simultaneously and contributed to the spread of SARS-related coronavirus in the Hong Kong residential estate of Amoy Gardens." [24]

However, epidemiologists continue to speculate as to whether contamination through floor drains and light wells is an adequate explanation for the outbreak. Stephen Ng, a researcher at the Chinese University of Hong Kong, has suggested that the rats at Amoy Gardens played an important role in the outbreak. Ng argues that the spatial distribution of the flats that were infected, as well as the different dates on which people fell ill, could be explained if the virus was spread by rats living in the estate. This hypothesis has yet to be tested.[25]

* * *

By the beginning of April, the doctors, nurses and nursing assistants who were at the front line of Hong Kong's health system were perilously close to breaking point. These were men and women who had been trained to heal and care for the sick. They had not been prepared for a situation where they would have to risk their lives and those of their families each time they went into work. Medical professionals who were accustomed to seeing sickness and death in others now had to cope with the knowledge that within a matter of hours, they too could become patients struggling with this illness. Peter Cameron, head of the Trauma and Emergency Centre at the Prince of Wales Hospital, described his experience in an article in the *Medical Journal of Australia*, "This is the first time I have felt threatened by the work I do. Perhaps it's a similar experience to that of a policeman on his first 'stakeout' when he realised he might get shot. As a doctor, you know you are potentially vulnerable to the getting of all sorts of illness, but rarely a devastating or life threatening one."[26]

The psychological pressures were increased by the isolation that most doctors and nurses faced in the course of their work. Many stayed away from their families, their natural source of support, by moving to hotels or sending family members abroad. In every family where there was a medical worker dealing with SARS, there were agonizing decisions to be made about how to keep loved ones safe. Osmond Kwok, the doctor with a practice in the Amoy Gardens area, recalled the discussions that he and his wife had on what the best course of action was for their two children, aged 10 and 14. "I could have sent them away, but we decided that they need support too. It's a mutual thing. If I send them away, I have lost their support and they lose support too." He and his wife decided that since neither she nor their children were going out at all, they were not really at risk. The only risk could come from Kwok himself, who was seeing SARS patients. So he, like other doctors throughout Hong Kong, devised an elaborate set of measures to ensure that he did not contaminate his family.[27]

As soon as he came home, the rest of the family would disappear into their rooms. He would strip just inside the entrance and go straight to the shower. After that, he would eat by himself, using crockery and utensils that were kept for his use only. Then, he would join his family in the living room, sitting a little apart from everyone else and turned away from them." I would just sit there, not talking much. Even when I did talk to the others, I would look away from them. I would sleep by myself, in a separate room." This was a new and uniquely stressful experience. "It was difficult, because even though you can see your family around you, you are really isolated. You see them, but you try not to talk to them. Everything had to be separate. I had my own telephone, my own car. That was the hard part. The isolation, you see people but you can't talk to them because it could be dangerous. And you don't see your friends and colleagues either, because that could be dangerous too."

As can be expected when men and women put their lives at risk and work under conditions they have not experienced before or been trained to deal with, fear, anger and recrimination often erupted. Doctors and nurses who were working long hours under potentially life-threatening conditions would vent their feelings and fears in newspaper interviews and radio talk shows, often complaining about their superiors. One nurse at Princess Margaret Hospital called into a radio show and broke down as she recounted the stress that she and her colleagues were under. Twenty doctors and nurses at the hospital had fallen ill, she said. "We've taken protective measures. I don't understand why we are falling ill," she added, echoing what other nurses and doctors working with SARS patients were feeling. "The doctors don't know how to treat us and we are at high risk."

Many medical professionals felt that they were not being given the right type of protective equipment. With supplies running low, several hospitals restricted the higher performance, but also more expensive, N95 masks to staff who were actually treating SARS patients, while other staff members were provided with ordinary surgical masks. Infection control experts would stress that with a disease like SARS, it is not high tech masks and other equipment that provide the maximum protection, but rather sticking to the basic rules of infection control — frequent washing of hands and showering, changing of masks and gowns whenever necessary to prevent cross-infection between patients and so on. Simple masks that were changed several times a day were more effective than more complicated masks that were often worn throughout the day, and were uncomfortable and difficult to breathe through.

Dr Seto Wing Hong, the head of infection control at Queen Mary Hospital, used daily newsletters to drill his staff on the effectiveness of hand washing and following basic techniques rather than relying on sophisticated suits and breathing equipment that had not been designed for hospital needs. "The basics are still the same. A good surgical mask, and if there are possibilities of aerosols generated, wear an N-95. Wash your hands after each patient contact. Be calm and avoid lapses. If you inadvertently contaminate yourself, wash, wash and wash immediately." But many of those on the frontlines were convinced that they needed specialized equipment if they were to survive. One nurse, a Miss Lam, phoned into a radio show to complain that she and her colleagues were only being issued surgical masks, as opposed to N95 masks, and that they were now at greater risk: "My colleagues and I are now at a loss as to what we are to do next."[28]

Hong Kong has a well-equipped, well-funded public hospital system that is probably as good as that found anywhere in the world. But SARS exposed a crucial weakness in the system: the lack of proper training in infection control. This was the first time in their careers that doctors and nurses were confronting a disease this contagious, and they were unprepared. Many hospital workers were unfamiliar with basic precautions such as how to wear a mask properly, not touching a mask with hands, gowning and de-gowning in the right way and wearing spectacles in front of masks rather than behind them. Even among those who did know better, working long hours under stressful conditions led to slip-ups, and this led to infection.

Though it took a while for overworked, overstressed doctors and nurses to realize it, by April the peak of the epidemic in Hong Kong was over. After the dramatic days at the end of March when there were 60 and 70 new cases coming in every day, the number of cases dropped in April to an average of around 35 new cases a day. The number of patients in hospital also gradually began to drop. From a peak of nearly 950 patients in hospital on April 17, the numbers gradually began to go down, as the numbers of patients being discharged from hospital after recovery began to outstrip the numbers of new cases coming in. The epidemic died down as public health authorities became better at getting people to hospital quickly before they could infect others. Transmission of the virus also slowed as people in Hong Kong instinctively changed their normal patterns of behaviour to avoid doing things that put them at risk of catching the disease. People stayed at home rather going to cinemas, restaurants and other public places where the virus could spread. Schools were closed, keeping children at home and closing off opportunities for a school-based epidemic.[29]

Tracing those people with whom SARS patients had been in contact was one of the most important aspects of controlling its spread. The Department of Health already had in place a well-established and tested system of contact tracing, which was originally developed to control tuberculosis. But the speed at which SARS progressed soon overwhelmed the system. As the number of cases mounted, and patient data came in from different hospitals, it became apparent that the information needed to be put into a centralized electronic database. This database could then be used to track patient numbers, trace contacts and provide an overall view of the geographic spread of the disease.

Information coming in from different hospitals was first entered into a centralized "eSARS" database. This was also linked to a police information system that helped locate and trace people who had been in close contact with SARS patients. The Hong Kong Police system was devised to solve a unique Hong Kong problem. A single address or name can be spoken and written in different ways in each of the three languages in use in the territory: Cantonese, Mandarin and English. The spoken name of a building or street could be completely different in each of these three languages, and so could the written name. The police computer system sorts and matches the names and addresses of buildings in all three languages, and helped public health authorities to locate geographic clusters of infection.

Nurses were trained to trace people who might have been in contact with SARS patients by asking the "three w's" — *who* had they been in contact with over the last ten days, *when* had contact occurred and *where* had it taken place. This information was then fed into the police system, and analyzed for geographical and other patterns of infection.

Getting sick people to hospital as soon as possible and isolating them from the rest of the community put a brake on the spread of the disease, and by the middle of May, the numbers of new cases coming into hospitals had come down into the single figures. By June, four months after the outbreak began, it was clear that the back of the epidemic had been broken. On June 2, one patient was admitted to hospital with SARS. And then there were no more. On June 23, after 20 days had passed since the last patient with SARS was admitted to hospital, the WHO declared that Hong Kong was no longer a place where SARS was transmitting locally.

4

A GLOBAL EMERGENCY

IT was 2.30 a.m. in Geneva and the telephone was ringing. Dr Michael J Ryan fumbled for the phone and mumbled a groggy greeting into the receiver. Seconds later, the burly Irish doctor was wide awake, all thought of sleep dispelled.[1]

The caller at the other end was from the Manila office of the World Health Organization (WHO), and his message was alarming. Flying over the Atlantic Ocean on a Singapore Airlines flight was a critically ill man who had to be hospitalized in an isolation ward as soon as possible. With him were his pregnant wife and his mother-in-law, who could be falling ill as well. There were over 300 passengers on the jet, which was bound for Singapore via Frankfurt, and unless the man was taken off the plane, they were all in danger.

Ryan, who was in charge of the WHO's Global Outbreak Alert and Response Network (GOARN), knew he had to act quickly. The man on the plane, Leong Hoe Nam, a 32-year-old infectious diseases specialist from Singapore, had probably caught the mysterious pneumonia-like disease that was spreading through Hong Kong, Vietnam, China and Singapore. Nobody knew what the disease was, what caused it or how to treat it. What was known was that the disease was highly contagious, and that its spread to new corners of the world had to be prevented at all cost.

The first priority was to get the doctor and his family off the aircraft, both for their safety, and to protect the other passengers. The worst case scenario would be if other passengers on the plane caught the disease and carried it to new parts of the world.

The flight was now on its way to Frankfurt. Ryan got on the phone and roused the German health authorities, impressing on them the severity of the situation. Given the way the new disease was spreading, the Germans needed no convincing. When the aircraft landed in Frankfurt, ambulances and medical personnel dressed in biological hazard suits were on hand to escort Leong, his wife and his mother-in-law to an isolation ward at the Frankfurt University's Medical School Hospital.

By the time Ryan got back into bed at 4 a.m. to try and catch some sleep, he knew he would have a long day ahead of him. The WHO had been lucky to have had prior warning about the sick doctor on the aircraft. But how long could it continue to be lucky? With hundreds of thousands of people travelling by plane every day, it was just a matter of time before other sick people unwittingly spread the disease. Something needed to be done quickly to alert doctors and health workers everywhere to this danger. If a patient with this new disease could walk into a clinic anywhere in the world, doctors needed to know what symptoms to look out for, and what to do about it.

It had already been a long hard fortnight for Ryan and his team of doctors and epidemiologists at GOARN. They were an experienced lot. In the two years since the unit had been established, they had responded to epidemics of Ebola in Uganda, yellow fever in West Africa, haemorrhagic fever in Afghanistan and a host of smaller outbreaks across the world. In the process, they had developed a well-oiled mechanism for dealing with diseases in remote corners of the world: flying in epidemiologists and laboratory teams, arranging for the delivery of medical supplies and equipment and working with local health authorities to improve infection control and prevent disease from spreading.

But this new disease already seemed unlike anything they had faced before. The crisis had begun earlier in the month with a worried message from one of their colleagues in Hanoi, Carlo Urbani. Urbani, a bearded, extroverted 46-year-old Italian physician, was the infectious diseases specialist at the WHO's Hanoi office and had responded to a call on February 28 from the Hanoi French Hospital, a small private hospital catering largely to the city's expatriate population. The doctors at the hospital were puzzled by the symptoms of a patient who had admitted himself a few days earlier, on February 26, with a fever, aching body and a dry cough. The man, Johnny Cheng, a Chinese-American and manager for a US textile company, had come to Hanoi to visit a garment factory, but had felt out of sorts since arriving from Hong Kong. His symptoms worsened at the hospital. His chest X-rays showed pneumonia-like patches, his fever was high and doctors found he was not responding to antibiotics.[2]

Cheng's condition deteriorated rapidly, and Urbani was alarmed by what he saw. He asked for blood and tissue samples to be sent to WHO-affiliated laboratories for testing, and reported back to his colleagues that they could be facing a particularly virulent kind of flu. Within days, doctors and nurses at the French Hospital began to catch the disease as well, and Urbani and his colleagues at the WHO office knew they were onto something unusual and dangerous. By the end of the week, 14 doctors and nurses at the French Hospital had come down with the illness, and there was panic in the hospital. Whatever this disease was, it did not respond to drugs, and the speed at which it spread and struck down young, healthy medical staff was terrifying.

Emails and telephone calls flew between the WHO's Hanoi office, the regional office in Manila and headquarters in Geneva as Urbani sent out the alert that an unusual and dangerous disease, characterized by a high rate of infection among doctors and nurses, had broken out in Vietnam. The disease had to be prevented from spreading out of the hospital environment into the community at large. Urbani and his boss Pascale Brudon, a 52-year-old Frenchwoman who headed the WHO office in Hanoi, requested urgent help to try and control the disease.

While the WHO was gearing up for emergency action in Vietnam, on March 11, a message arrived at the WHO headquarters in Geneva from the Health Department in Hong Kong regarding an alarming outbreak of respiratory illness among hospital staff at the Prince of Wales Hospital. The descriptions of the illness in Hong Kong, as well as the way it was affecting hospital staff, suggested that Hong Kong and Hanoi had been hit by the same epidemic. The disease also seemed suspiciously similar to that mentioned in reports the WHO had received in February from the Chinese government regarding an outbreak in Guangdong province. There too, the disease had hit health care workers disproportionately.

After the news from Hong Kong came in, Ryan's boss, David Heymann, a veteran epidemiologist who headed the WHO's infectious diseases unit, decided there was no time to be lost. The world had to be warned about this new disease. On March 12, the WHO put out a global alert describing the symptoms of this severe pneumonia and recommending that patients suspected of having the disease be placed in isolation.[3]

Later that day, halfway across the world, Allison McGeer, an infection control specialist at Mount Sinai Hospital in Toronto, Canada, saw the WHO warning about the new disease. The next day, March 13, she got a call from a doctor asking for advice about three members of a family who had come down with a particularly severe form of pneumonia that did not seem to be responding to treatment. When

McGeer learned that the elderly mother of the family had died a few days earlier after catching a flu-like illness during a holiday in Hong Kong, she put two and two together and alerted her colleagues that the new disease had probably reached Canada.[4]

At around the same time, Singapore public health officials realized that the symptoms of three young women who had been hospitalized with an unusual pneumonia they had caught after a shopping trip to Hong Kong in late February matched the WHO's case description for the new disease. One of the women, who had been in hospital since March 1, had already passed on the disease to five other people, and by March 14, Singapore had nine cases.[5]

In Geneva, David Heymann summoned his team to an emergency meeting at 6 a.m., just hours after the sick doctor had been taken off the flight in Frankfurt and put in isolation. In Heymann's mind there was little doubt about what needed to be done: the WHO had to put out an even stronger message in the form of an emergency travel alert warning airlines, travellers and doctors around the world about the disease. And it needed to be done immediately. As Heymann recalled, "We had a disease that was spreading internationally, we had no cause for the disease, we thought it was infectious, no vaccine, no drugs. We had no choice but to act." [6]

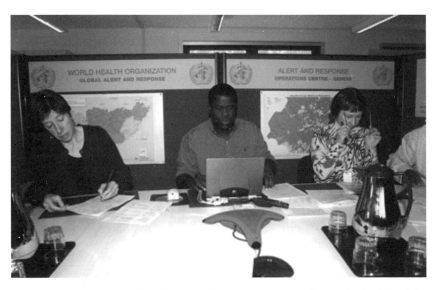

WHO SARS team at work at the control room in Geneva during the height of the crisis. (P. Virot: WHO)

In the WHO though, as in any other intergovernmental organization with 192 governments as members, the words "rapid" and "action" rarely go together. Decisions tend to be the end product of years of ponderous debate in which each government tries to ensure that its own interests are protected. Not surprisingly, these decisions are often little more than a string of compromises expressed in an impenetrably worded official resolution.

But on this day, things had to be done differently. People were dying of an unknown disease that was creeping across the world and the WHO could not afford to wait to consult with all its member governments. It had to take the most direct route and warn the world about the situation.

In doing so, Heymann and his team were taking risks. For one, governments do not like it when international organizations take matters into their own hands and communicate directly with their citizens without first telling them. The WHO might well have found itself the recipient of irate phone calls from ministries of health all over the world, asking why the organization was spreading unnecessary panic.

A greater risk was that the WHO knew next to nothing about the disease except that it was a severe respiratory illness that appeared to be spreading internationally. But what if the outbreaks in Hong Kong and Hanoi were completely separate diseases? Even if it was the same disease, the WHO had so little data that there was very little it could tell doctors. What if the disease later turned out not to be as serious as it seemed? As a respected scientific agency, could the WHO take the risk of crying wolf?

"We really had to take our hearts in our hands," recalled Ryan. "We might have been making associations between things that might not have been associated. We had only a handful of cases, we had no laboratory data to support a new, unknown disease. So it really came down to that balance between pulling the trigger and telling the world we have a new disease, and the risk that we might be wrong."[7]

The people sitting around the meeting table at the WHO's headquarters that morning were not typical international civil servants. They were epidemiologists who had been out in the field and stared disease in the face. Heymann, a veteran of the smallpox eradication campaign, had tramped through the villages of eastern India vaccinating people, and had searched for the origins of Ebola in the jungles of West Africa. Guenael Rodier, Heymann's deputy, had been in the thick of Ebola outbreaks, as had Mike Ryan. It was this knowledge of what a

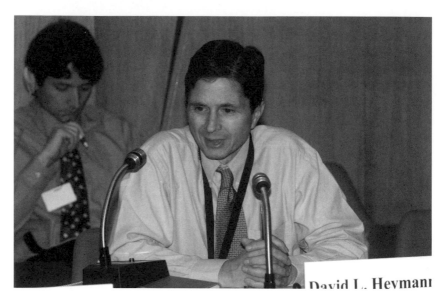

David Heymann, leader of the WHO's SARS team at a press conference in Geneva. (P. Virot: WHO)

disease could do if allowed to rampage unchecked that weighed on them and persuaded them of the need to act quickly, despite political and institutional obstacles.

Heymann had a powerful ally backing him in the form of Gro Harlem Brundtland, the Director-General of the WHO. One of her senior advisers, Denis Aitken, was at the early morning session, listening while Heymann and his team set out their case for urgent action and keeping Brundtland updated on the discussion. By noon the global alert had been drafted. Everything now hinged on whether Brundtland would give it the go-ahead.

In her five years as Director-General, Brundtland, a former prime minister of Norway, had brought a Scandinavian directness to the workings of the WHO, shaking up the organization and radically changing the way in which it worked. When SARS broke out, she had just four months to go before she retired from office. In the final days of her tenure, rather than risk controversy and the ire of member governments, the normal bureaucratic proceeding would have been to ask Heymann's team to wait a few days or weeks until more was known about the disease.

But to the team's great relief, Brundtland backed their decision to issue an immediate alert. As she saw it, this was the right thing to do.

Here was a new disease that had struck down a great many people, and which was clearly more than just a simple cold or flu. Within a few weeks it had already spread all over the world. Without a cure, the only step that could be taken was to stop transmission of the disease by making people aware of it. If people were not aware of the disease, it could spread further. In addition, Brundtland did not want the WHO to be blamed later for not having alerted the world to a new disease that needed urgent attention.[8]

Her staff admired her decision to back them. Mike Ryan considered it a brave decision: "She was coming to the end of her tenure, and the last thing she would want to do was to go out crying wolf to the world. For her politically, she took a huge risk."[9]

That morning, as they worked towards a deadline of noon to get the global alert out, Heymann's team suddenly realized that they did not have a name for the new disease. "What are we going to call it?" asked Dick Thompson, a veteran *Time* magazine science writer who had joined the WHO as a communication officer. Heymann was clear that the name they chose should not draw attention to any particular city or geographical area. "We did not want to stigmatise particular areas, it could not be called Hong Kong flu or Hanoi flu," he said. After kicking around different options, they came up with SARS, a sibilant acronym that would soon be echoing around the world.

SARS, or Severe Acute Respiratory Syndrome, was as neutral a description of the disease as was possible and described its most striking clinical feature. But despite their efforts, the WHO team did not quite succeed in finding a name that avoided the stigma associated with geographical reference. What none of them realized at the time was that SARS was unfortunately close to the three-letter acronym SAR, or Special Administrative Region, by which Hong Kong was known officially. In the weeks that followed, as Hong Kong struggled to shake off its plague-ridden image, many in the territory would regard the name of the disease as another cruel twist of fate. The Hong Kong government was at first reluctant to refer to the disease as SARS, and called it by the more imprecise but politically palatable term, "atypical pneumonia."

The announcement that went out that Saturday morning was a wake-up call.[10] The international agency charged with safeguarding global health was telling the world that a new disease without a cure was at loose and spreading across the world at the speed of modern jet travel. The emergency advisory included a message from Brundtland that summed up what the WHO was trying to say: "This syndrome,

SARS, is now a worldwide health threat. The world needs to work together to find its cause, cure the sick, and stop its spread."

Given the speed at which SARS was travelling, it was clear to everyone at the WHO, from Brundtland on down, that the epidemic had to be fought internationally as well as locally. It was not enough for doctors, nurses and public health officials to fight SARS in their own hospitals and communities. All these efforts had to be coordinated, and help had to be rushed to countries that were not able to stop the disease from spreading. If SARS was to be controlled, it had to be controlled across the world at the same time. If there was even a single weak link in the chain of containment, it would be impossible to stamp out the disease.

In those early days, everyone at the WHO headquarters suspected that there was such a weak link, in a country to which they had frustratingly little access: China. As will be discussed later, a great deal of time and diplomatic effort was spent penetrating the wall of Chinese bureaucracy and integrating the fight against SARS in China with what was going on in other parts of the world.

But in those feverish days in March in Geneva, as the WHO grappled with this strange new disease that had leaped up out of nowhere and grabbed the world by the throat, the first priority was to rush resources and aid to countries that needed it, and to collect information about the disease from across the world so that this could be shared.

Leaving China aside, Vietnam was an urgent priority. Vietnam was the poorest of the countries where SARS had broken out, and its public health system had the fewest resources. Urbani and Pascale Brudon decided that the Vietnamese government had to be made aware of how serious this new disease was, and of the importance of urgent action to prevent it from spreading in the community. On March 9, Urbani and Brudon had a four-hour meeting with the Vietnamese Vice Minister of Health, Nguyen Van Thuong, and other health officials at which Urbani made a presentation urging that strict infection control measures be put in place to stop the disease from spreading in the community, and that international experts be allowed in to study the disease and help stop its spread. Nguyen Van Thuong, the Vice Minister, was convinced and threw his weight behind Urbani's recommendations. Within days an international team had arrived to help local doctors. The French Hospital was quarantined, infection control measures were tightened and contact tracing was put in place to identify potential carriers of the disease.[11] This swift early action by the Vietnamese government paid off. On April 28, a little over two months after Johnny Cheng was admitted to the French Hospital, the spread of SARS in the country had been stopped. Vietnam was the first SARS-affected country to achieve this level of control.

But before the success in Vietnam, there were weeks of exhaustion, frayed nerves and a seemingly constant stream of setbacks that David Heymann and his team had to face, including the death of one of their own. Carlo Urbani, the man who had alerted the world to SARS and had spent countless days and nights with patients, doctors and nurses helping them to control the disease, was ultimately struck down by the disease.

On March 11, Urbani took a break from his work with SARS patients and set off for Bangkok for a conference on parasitic diseases, his area of speciality. But before leaving Hanoi, he began to feel ill and spoke to his boss Pascale Brudon, who thought it was probably exhaustion and urged him to go. However, she took the precaution of warning her colleagues at the WHO office in Bangkok that Urbani was not well and might need help. When Urbani landed at Bangkok airport that night, Scott Dowell, an epidemiologist at the US Center for Diseases Control (CDC) was waiting for him. Urbani had felt increasingly ill on the flight, and asked to be hospitalized in an isolation ward. Eighteen days later he would die from the disease he had brought to the world's notice.[12]

Carlo Urbani had been a larger than life character with passions ranging from organ music to piloting light aircraft. His real passion though was treating diseases in the developing countries, particularly parasitic diseases that were easy to prevent but took huge tolls, particularly among children. This work had taken him from Mauritania, where he was the first to document the way a parasitical infection, *Schistosoma mansoni*, was transmitted, to the Maldives and the Mekong Delta, where he tracked hookworm and flatworm infections. In the two years he had been with the WHO in Hanoi, Urbani had worked on finding cost-effective ways to control parasitic worms.[13]

In between stints with the WHO, Urbani had also worked with the medical charity Medecins Sans Frontieres (MSF), and had founded an Italian chapter of the organization. It was as president of MSF Italy that Urbani had been invited to Norway in 1999 to receive the Nobel Peace Prize on behalf of MSF. A close friend at the WHO, Lorenzo Savioli, recalled that a few days before he fell ill, Urbani' s wife Giuliani had urged him to stop spending so much time with highly infectious patients and think of their three children, aged between 4 and 17. Urbani's reply was typical: "If I can't work in such situations what am I here for?

Answering e-mails, going to cocktails and pushing paper?"[14] Urbani knew the risks he was taking with a disease as infectious as SARS, but like so many of the other doctors who would succumb to the illness, he pushed on, treating patients until he could no longer do so.

Urbani's death at the end of March was only the latest blow in a war that health experts just did not seem to be winning. Every day seemed to bring fresh bad news. The outbreak of SARS in the Amoy Gardens housing estate in Hong Kong just days before had raised worries that SARS might be transmitting through the environment, rather than only through close personal contact. If this was the case, the WHO team knew they might be looking at an unstoppable worldwide epidemic. As the number of cases in Hong Kong continued to mount, there were real worries that the hospital system there would become swamped, and that patients would decide to go elsewhere for treatment, taking the disease with them.

From Vietnam there was the disturbing news that two cases of SARS had turned up in the provinces outside Hanoi, indicating that the disease might be loose in the countryside. From Singapore there was news of an unexplained cluster of patients who did not seem to have gotten the disease from any known source. If so, was the disease spreading in some new and inexplicable way?

Whatever the WHO and public health officials around the world did, nothing seemed to stop the inexorable spread of the disease. On March 12, when the first alert was sounded, there were 55 cases from Hong Kong and Hanoi. Within a month, there were 3000 cases and more than 100 deaths in 20 countries and on every continent. By the end of the first week of May, there were 7000 cases being reported in 30 countries. The beginning of May was the peak of worldwide outbreak, with 200 new cases being reported a day, mainly from China. "There seemed to be no end in sight," said Dick Thompson of those stress-filled days. "We were all working at least 15 hours a day, day after day, and it just seemed to go on. Then Carlo died, and that was really traumatic."[15]

Thompson's own day of answering questions from the media would begin around 3 a.m. Geneva time, when the first phone calls would start coming in from journalists in Hong Kong. He would go into work for an 8 a.m. strategy meeting, and continue to answer calls until late in the night, when US and Canadian journalists began their working day. In between there would be hundreds of emails to answer and press releases to draft. "I would get messages about all sorts of things. I had one from a person in Prague asking whether it was safe to travel to

Paris," he recalled. "Everyone was working seven days a week, we were all physically exhausted, and afraid as well. We did not know where this disease was going next."

Trying to stop the disease from going anywhere new was crucial to the WHO's strategy for containing SARS. The only way to do this was to ensure that the risk of spreading SARS through airline travel was minimized. The ability of a single sick patient on an airplane to spread the disease was illustrated by the case of an Air China flight from Hong Kong to Beijing. On March 15, while David Heymann and his team were toiling away on their global travel alert in Geneva, a 72-year-old man boarded Air China flight 112 from Hong Kong to Beijing. The elderly man was going back home after a visit to see family in Hong Kong. In Hong Kong, he had visited a sick niece at the Prince of Wales Hospital, where he had been infected with the SARS virus.

By the time he got on the flight back to Beijing, the old man was clearly ill. Not only was he sick, he also happened to be a super-spreader of the disease. From his seat, 14E, he infected 21 other passengers and crew members, some sitting as far as seven seats away from him. Two stewardesses on the flight, Meng Chunyung and Fan Jingling, caught the virus and took it back to their homes in Mongolia, setting off a chain of nearly 300 infections in the province. Meng, 27, passed the disease on to her husband Li Ling, who later died, as well as to her mother, father, brother and doctor. A *New York Times* reporter who caught up with her in hospital in Huhhot, the Inner Mongolian capital, found her distraught. "I never imagined that this kind of tragedy would fall on me and my family and take away the person dearest to me," she said.[16]

Four Taiwanese employees of a Taipei-based engineering firm also on the flight would catch the virus and fall sick in Taiwan. One Singaporean woman would add to the number of cases in Singapore. Also on board were a group of 35 tourists from Hong Kong who were going to spend a week in Beijing. On their return to Hong Kong, at least 10 of them fell ill with SARS, setting off a frantic attempt by the Hong Kong Department of Health to contact all the other passengers and crew on the fateful flight to warn them of the danger.

The legacy of flight CA 112 would spread internationally as well. One of the passengers infected was an official in the Chinese Ministry of Commerce. He would later fly to Bangkok for a conference, where he would feel the first symptoms of SARS. Sitting next to him on his return flight to Beijing on March 23 would be Pekka Aro, a 52-year-old Finnish official at the International Labour Organization (ILO) in

Geneva. Aro, who was travelling to Beijing to prepare for a China Employment Forum jointly organized by the ILO and the Chinese government, would fall ill five days later on March 28, and would be hospitalized on April 2. Four days later he would become the first foreigner to die of SARS in China.

The way SARS spread from this single infected airline passenger was unusual.[17] While infected travellers could and did spread the disease to far flung destinations, they rarely did so during the actual course of a flight. It was once they got to the other end that they tended to spread the virus. Modern aircraft use HEPA (high-efficiency particulate air) filters, the same kind of filters that are used in hospital operating theatres and emergency rooms, to clean the air in an aircraft cabin. These filters can trap and clean coronavirus-laden sneezes. The only risk is sitting next to, or a couple of rows directly in front of or behind an infected person coughing up germs.

During the five months that SARS was spreading actively in different countries, only 27 people were estimated to have been infected during the course of an airline flight, and 22 of them were on flight CA 112. No one has a clear idea of why the disease spread so widely on that one flight. Fortunately, this proved to be the exception rather than the rule.[18]

But at the time, no one could be sure that the disease would not spread on aircraft. For the WHO in Geneva, incidents like flight CA 112 were proof that more needed to be done to ensure that people with SARS were not boarding international flights. The only way to do this was to ask airports and airline staff to check passengers for any of the outward symptoms of SARS: fever, a cough or recent close contact with SARS patients. On March 27, the WHO put out a recommendation that airline passengers from the five areas that were known to be SARS-affected: Hong Kong, Singapore, Hanoi, China's Guangdong province and Taiwan, be screened at airports before departure using a simple questionnaire asking whether they had any of the symptoms of SARS.

In the weeks that followed, Singapore and Hong Kong would find high tech solutions to the problem of screening passengers, and install sophisticated temperature scanners that would check passengers for fever, much like the metal detecting barriers that are standard in all international airports. Soon other airports around the world began doing the same, and just as metal detectors became standard more than a decade ago, when aircraft hijacking was a major threat to security, temperature screens are becoming standard in airports today, reflecting the latest threat to human security: disease.

Despite the array of modern technology available to fight disease, as the WHO developed its strategy for fighting SARS, it became apparent that the real key to containing the epidemic was to use one of the oldest weapons against disease: isolating and quarantining sick people to prevent them from spreading disease to others. When the bubonic plague swept through Europe from Central Asia in the thirteenth century, cities like Venice protected themselves through the simple expedient of forcing ships and travellers to wait outside the city for 40 days before coming in. The city authorities judged correctly that anyone carrying the disease would die within that period, and that anyone who was alive would not be carrying the plague.

Since then, modern medicine has given us vaccinations to prevent diseases, and powerful drugs to treat them. But in the case of a new disease like SARS, there were neither vaccines nor drugs to rely on. The only effective way of stopping SARS from spreading was tracking down sick people and preventing them from infecting others.

To back up the basic public health strategy of isolating sick people, the WHO harnessed the power of modern technology to create an innovative virtual network of laboratories and doctors across the world to pool experience and findings. When SARS broke out, microbiologists, epidemiologists and clinicians in labs all over the world began working on the same set of questions: what causes this disease, how does it spread and how do we treat it?

Normally, these laboratories would have worked independently. Even though scientific research is at heart a collaborative effort, researchers and the labs they belong to are extremely reluctant to collaborate with each other. Human egos and the realities of scientific funding combine to ensure that cutthroat competition rather than selfless collaboration is the norm in scientific endeavour. Scientists, as much as athletes or investment bankers, want to be the best in their field. The kudos go to those who make the big discoveries and publish papers first. Not to those who come in second by confirming other people's findings. And it is not a question of ego alone. The research grants on which both science and scientists depend for their survival tend to go to those who make the big discoveries and publish first in prestigious scientific journals. There are few prizes in science for coming in second.

Perhaps the WHO's most singular achievement in those early crisis-filled days was to persuade some of the biggest names in virology to put aside any individual ambition to become the first to discover the agent causing this new disease, and to pool their findings in the interests

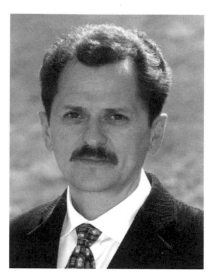

Klaus Stohr, coordinator of the WHO's global laboratory network. (P. Virot: WHO)

of getting an answer as quickly as possible. It fell to Klaus Stohr, a German virologist who headed the WHO's global influenza programme, to cobble together a coalition of the world's best known laboratories and researchers to work together to crack the puzzle of what was causing SARS. Stohr, a veterinarian by training, had been running the influenza programme since 2001, and had put together a global network of influenza research laboratories. The personal contacts as well as the diplomatic skills he had acquired in creating this network were to serve him well as he worked to create a virtual network to identify the organism causing SARS.

On Saturday and Sunday, March 15 and 16, after David Heymann's team had sent out the WHO global travel warning, Stohr got on the phone with the leading laboratories around the world, many of which had already begun working on SARS, and persuaded them to work together. He set out the ground rules: the WHO would put up a secure website where each lab could post its findings, whether these were electron microscope pictures, viral gene sequences or the results of diagnostic tests. Laboratories would share samples, analyze them using different techniques and then share the results.[19]

The researchers would talk to each other every day through a teleconference at 1 p.m. Geneva time, and share their findings with their colleagues. Given the competitive nature of the scientists involved, Stohr convinced them to agree that all data would be kept confidential, and that no lab or researcher would use someone else's findings without prior permission.

All of the 11 labs Stohr approached — ranging from the giant Centre for Diseases Control and Prevention (CDC) in Atlanta, to the three small labs in Hong Kong at the Hong Kong and Chinese Universities and the Government Virus Unit —came on board.

On March 17, the labs held their first teleconference with Klaus Stohr moderating from Geneva. In what would become a standard routine, Stohr went from participant to participant, asking them what they had to report, and then set an informal agenda by which different laboratories would divide the work to be done between them, rather than duplicating each other's efforts. Stohr also ensured that samples would be shared between laboratories.

In the weeks that followed, it would become clear that this novel approach to science was a definite improvement on the earlier pattern of laboratories working in isolation. One lab's findings could be followed up almost instantly by other researchers and either confirmed or rejected. Samples could be shared and work divided between laboratories. While the WHO paid tribute to the selflessness of the various participating laboratories, in reality the old competitive habits died hard. Several of the laboratories felt that the CDC, the largest of the laboratories, and arguably the most competitive, was not as open as other laboratories. Participants noted that after a while, the CDC kept a low profile in the daily teleconferences, listening in but not contributing much. "The CDC seemed to drop out of the conferences, and the others noticed it. It took a lot of diplomacy to persuade everyone to stay in," observed Dick Thompson, the WHO communication officer.[20]

The conflicting pulls of the need to collaborate in controlling a global epidemic before it got out of control, and the desire of individual laboratories and researchers to go down in the record books as the first to discover the causal agent for SARS surfaced again once the coronavirus had been identified as the cause of the disease. The CDC suggested that it had been the first to do so, with other laboratories confirming the CDC's findings. The record however, showed that it was the Hong Kong University team that made the initial breakthrough.

Also, despite the initial understanding that all research would be collaborative, when the time came to publish, each team raced ahead to be the first to publish its findings. The WHO had hoped to publish a single scientific article in the names of all the participating laboratories. The CDC however, said that it was going to publish its findings in the *New England Journal of Medicine*. A team of German researchers did the same, and the Hong Kong University team published its findings in the *Lancet*, a few days ahead of the others.

The laboratory network that Stohr had put together was soon followed by a network of epidemiologists and clinicians coordinated by Mark Salter, a British doctor who had been seconded to the WHO. These networks allowed the WHO to put together and make sense of the information being gathered all over the world on the way the disease was spreading, what kinds of treatment were showing the best results and the hundreds of other questions that needed to be answered to make sense of SARS.

In two cramped rooms on the fourth and fifth floors of an annex to the WHO's main headquarters, researchers spent 15- and 16-hour days gathering data, entering it into computers and analyzing it. Were there cases of people catching SARS in unexplained ways? Were there any hospital practices that seemed to be working particularly well in controlling the spread of infection among doctors and nurses? Were there other clinical practices that needed to be avoided at all costs? These were the kinds of questions that needed urgent answers if SARS was to be fought effectively. And the only way to get those answers was for the WHO team to gather every scrap of information it could from hospitals and doctors fighting the disease all over the world, put it all together and then pass these findings back to the disease fighters on the ground.

As the data began to come in from SARS-afflicted regions across the world, there was one gaping hole that was increasingly impossible to ignore: China. In those hectic days in March and April, as SARS rampaged through Hong Kong, Singapore and Toronto and popped up in new cities on an almost daily basis, it was vital to find out what was happening in China. China was after all where it had all started in the late autumn of 2002, and it was there that the clues to the origins of SARS were to be found. It was also in China that the battle to stamp out this particular epidemic of SARS had to be fought. It did not matter if SARS was eliminated everywhere else in the world; as long as the disease continued to smoulder in the world's most populous nation, it was only a matter of time before it would erupt out into the rest of the world.

But getting information out of China was proving to be a dangerously slow exercise, and the longer it took, the more lives were put at risk in China as well as elsewhere. For the WHO and for the world at large, integrating China into the global disease-fighting effort became of the highest priority.

* * *

On February 23, 2003, Hitoshi Oshitani, a Japanese flu expert at the WHO's regional headquarters in Manila, and Keiji Fukuda, an influenza specialist at the CDC in Atlanta, flew into Beijing in what would be the first attempt by the WHO to send its experts into Guangdong province.

It was no coincidence that both men were influenza experts. By the end of February, the WHO had become increasingly suspicious that the illness in Guangdong was a particularly virulent form of influenza. Perhaps it was the "big one" that every influenza expert across the world had been watching out for: a mutant flu virus many times more virulent than normal, and to which few people in the world would have any natural immunity. If such a virus had emerged, the rest of the world had to be alerted as soon as possible, and new vaccines had to be developed to prevent a pandemic in which tens of millions might die.

Since December 2002, reports of a severe pneumonia-like disease had begun reaching the WHO headquarters. The Canadian Global Public Health Intelligence Network (GPHIN), a media tracking programme used by the WHO since 1997 to trawl through websites looking for news of disease outbreaks, had picked up newspaper reports from Guangdong about the outbreak there. The son of a retired WHO official travelling through China had also emailed his father about reports of a disease that was causing alarm in southern China, and this news had been passed on to the WHO.

Then the pharmaceutical company Roche unwittingly set off a whole series of alarms at the WHO. On February 9, the company's Chinese subsidiary held a press conference in Guangzhou at which company officials appeared to be saying that the new disease was similar to the disease responsible for the bird flu outbreak in Hong Kong in 1997, and that Roche's anti-flu drug, Tamiflu, was effective against it. The company was later forced to apologize for these claims, but when the report reached the WHO, it was another hint that a new flu virus might be on the loose.[21]

Dr Shigeru Omi, the head of the WHO's regional office in Manila, acted quickly and sent a formal request to the Chinese Ministry of Health on March 10 asking for more information about the pneumonia in Guangdong. The Ministry of Health reported back the next day that there had been 305 cases and 5 deaths in an outbreak of "atypical pneumonia" in six municipalities of Guangdong province, but stressed that the outbreak had ended. Health officials said that 105 of the cases were health care workers, while the remaining cases were household contacts of patients. The WHO, anxious to determine whether this was a new influenza outbreak, asked for more details of the cases. Three days later, on February 14, the Ministry of Health reported that the symptoms included high fever, a dry cough and muscular pains, and that the disease was clinically consistent with atypical pneumonia. There was no evidence that this was a flu outbreak.

While the WHO was mulling this over, an event in Hong Kong seemed to confirm initial fears that a new kind of influenza was raging in southern China. On February 19, a 33-year-old man died in Hong Kong after being infected by an avian influenza virus. At first it was believed that he had caught the disease on a visit to Guangdong. This was later found to be wrong — he had in fact been travelling in Fujian province, further to the east, when he fell ill. But the possibility that the disease might have come from Guangdong increased the probability that a new form of flu capable of causing a global pandemic was raging in southern China.

It became imperative to try and get more information from Guangdong, if only to rule out the possibility that this was a lethal new flu. The WHO was particularly anxious to get blood samples and throat swabs from patients that could be tested for the presence of the H5N1 avian flu virus or any related flu viruses. Chinese health officials had earlier assured the WHO that they had found no traces of flu, but WHO officials needed to be sure. "The Chinese health authorities had done quite a good investigation, and they were telling us that this was not influenza," Mike Ryan recalled. "But we were saying this could be a new strain, could we provide you with reagents, a new strain is not easy to identify. They were saying we've identified chlamydia, and we were saying we would like to check for flu."[22]

While these exchanges went back and forth, Shigeru Omi, the head of the WHO's regional office in Manila, wrote once again to the Ministry of Health in Beijing on February 20, the day after the bird flu death in Hong Kong, asking for permission to send a team to Guangzhou to investigate the outbreak. Omi had an ally in Tommy Thompson, the US Secretary of Health. Influenza preparedness is a major plank of US government health policy, and the country's main health protection agency, the CDC in Atlanta, had alerted the Department of Health and Human Services about the H5N1-related deaths in Hong Kong. Thompson made use of the visit to Washington DC by the Chinese Deputy Health Minister to press for permission for an international team of investigators to visit China.

The Chinese government gave permission for the visit, and Oshitani and Fukuda flew to Beijing. When they arrived, they found that while they were welcome in Beijing, they had no invitation to go to Guangdong from the provincial authorities there. The two researchers received briefings from the Chinese Ministry of Health, but there was little headway being made in getting to Guangdong. The provincial health authorities did not see any reason to have outside investigators come to Guangdong to look for bird flu when their own researchers had found no evidence of influenza. The Chinese also did not appear to be in any mood to allow a US investigator to wander around Guangzhou.

After receiving routine briefings in Beijing and spending two weeks waiting for permission to visit Guangdong, both Oshitani and Fukuda left in frustration. Their mission to Beijing was the first of several attempts by the WHO to penetrate China and gather information about how SARS had originated, how it was being treated and whether it was being brought under control in China.

The WHO's approach to getting China to open up was patient diplomacy. The WHO office in Beijing, headed by Henk Bekedam, a large, genial Dutchman with degrees in economics as well as in medicine, had been working to build relationships with officials at China's Ministry of Health, slowly persuading them of the necessity of providing more information to the WHO.

While this diplomacy would ultimately pay off, the process was slow. As seen earlier, China had just undergone a major transition in leadership. In this period of uncertainty, Chinese officials were not about to stick their necks out and agree to unusual WHO requests. The official line was clear: the outbreak in Guangdong was under control, it was not avian flu and it was probably a chlamydia infection. There was also no evidence that the disease spreading across the world was linked to the pneumonia in Guangdong, so perhaps the WHO was barking up the wrong tree. This was the sum and substance of the Chinese message.

A flavour of the exchanges between the WHO office in Beijing and the Chinese Ministry of Health was revealed in a report in the official *China Daily* newspaper of a meeting between Henk Bekedam and Health Minister Zhang Wenkang on March 19. Bekedam briefed Zhang on the spread of SARS overseas and asked for greater cooperation from China to prevent and control the disease. Zhang responded that he would be happy to expand cooperation with the WHO, but stressed that the "atypical pneumonia outbreak has been contained." He added that "pneumonia patients had recovered and the daily lives of local residents had returned to normal."[23]

But figures that the Chinese government would itself release a week later on March 26 would show that SARS was clearly not contained. At that time, the Ministry of Health told the WHO that 792 cases and 31 deaths had been reported in Guangdong province between November 16, 2002, when the first case was reported, and the end of February 2003. Earlier figures had indicated 305 cases between November and February 9. Some of the additional 387 cases could represent cases that had occurred earlier but were only now being classified as SARS. But even if this were the case, at least several hundred cases had occurred in Guangdong in the second half of February, indicating the disease was alive, kicking and spreading.

It was these rapid about turns, from soothing initial assurances that SARS was under control, to statistics that revealed quite the opposite, that created widespread doubts about the reliability of Chinese data, and suspicion that China was deliberately covering up the scale of the epidemic. But despite the fuzziness of what was being said in public, a combination of external pressures, as well as the realization within the Chinese government that SARS would cripple the country unless it was brought under control, forced China to gradually open up.

On Thursday, March 10, the WHO's Beijing office received the first official request from the Chinese government for assistance to investigate the Guangdong outbreak. Alan Schnur, the number two in the office, put together a list of experts who would be able to help. Ten days later, on March 23, a team of five international experts arrived in Beijing on a ground-breaking visit that would help create the conditions for the free flow of information from China.

But even after the WHO team arrived, the pace of progress was slow. And as SARS gathered strength, and as the number of cases worldwide continued to rise, the need for answers from China became more and more urgent. There was also a fundamental question to which a definitive answer was needed: was the disease that had been called "atypical pneumonia" in China the same disease that the rest of the world was calling SARS?

If in fact SARS was the Guangdong atypical pneumonia, as was strongly suspected, then the clinical experience in Guangdong would be of immense relevance to doctors the world over battling the disease. Cooperation from China would also make it possible to compare the coronavirus that was causing the outbreak in China with that in other parts of the world to see if the virus was mutating in any way. This in turn would help to determine whether the transmission characteristics of the disease or its virulence were changing. Above all, if this was the same disease, it was vital that China begin urgent efforts to stop its spread within the country. If SARS became endemic in the world's most populous nation, there was no way that it could be prevented from taking root in other parts of the world as well. But even though the WHO team had arrived in Beijing, they had still not received permission to visit Guangdong and collect the data they needed to answer basic questions about SARS.

In Geneva, Gro Harlem Brundtland was making her frustration with the speed of the Chinese response evident. The WHO office in Beijing was continuing to urge patience and citing the progress that had been made so far in building cooperation despite the political uncertainty caused by the leadership changes. Brundtland felt that they were giving China too much time, and that perhaps a direct approach by her to the new leadership in China would be a quicker approach. In an interview recorded as part of an internal WHO oral history of SARS, Brundtland revealed her feelings at the time. "I felt in our own internal discussions we were taking too much time, giving time to China, hoping they would respond next week maybe over the weekend, and I was feeling impatient about the patience on the part of our team, and in fact of the regional office and the country office."[24]

Bekedam's team was working on the Chinese Ministry of Health, trying to impress on officials the urgency of the situation. Brundtland in the end bowed to this approach, but in retrospect she was certain that if she had taken a more direct route and contacted the Chinese leadership directly, this could well have saved several weeks. "I know that we maybe could have saved two weeks, two and a half weeks by pushing it directly to a higher level from my side, or by going via the Chinese embassy here in Geneva."[25]

The pressure was however mounting on Brundtland to say something publicly about China's tardiness. On April 9, while in India to launch a polio control campaign, the WHO Director-General bluntly accused China of not cooperating with the WHO. "It would have been better if the Chinese government had been more open in the early stages, from November to March," she told the press. "We were asking questions, wanting to send in experts to help identify the source. It took too long before they felt the need to be helped. Next time something strange and new comes ... let us come in as soon as possible."[26]

It is a rare moment when the head of an intergovernmental organization criticizes one of its leading member states, and Brundtland's remarks clearly came as a shock to China, but whether this sped up the shift in Chinese attitudes is debatable. By the time Brundtland spoke out, the big decision had already been made in Beijing to cooperate with the WHO. The first WHO team had in fact arrived in Guangdong several days earlier, and was getting ready to prepare a report on its findings to submit to the Chinese government.

Brundtland's decision to speak out appears to have reflected her shrewd politician's instinct to let the world know that the WHO was willing to speak its mind, and was not simply sitting back and doing nothing in the face of China's slow response to the situation. She revealed her reasoning in an interview in June 2003, shortly before she retired from the WHO. "Why did I speak out? This was because when everybody among the journalists knew that weeks had passed while the disease was spreading in China, and they knew that WHO had not got the reports, there was no way to make as if that was not the case. Much better then to be straightforward and to explain that yes, China was too late in responding. I think that was best for everyone. For WHO and for China."[27]

The Chinese turn around was a result of a complex set of factors. On the one hand there was growing international pressure, from the WHO, but also from the US and other Western countries, urging China to reveal whatever it knew about the disease. The US Secretary of Health, Tommy Thompson, had a 45-minute telephone conversation with his counterpart Zhang Wenkang on April 4, urging the need for international cooperation to halt the spread of SARS. According to US officials, Zhang was receptive, but maintained that the disease had already peaked in Guangzhou, and that China was working to manage the outbreak. A press release by the US Health and Human Services Department on this conversation quoted Thompson as saying, "the minister of health was very cooperative" and that he wanted to do more with the US.[28]

The telephone conversation, promising though it appeared at the time, evidently did not achieve the results the US wanted, and two weeks later, at a European Union meeting in Rome, Thompson too would publicly criticize China for its lack of transparency. "We've been very upset at this lack of transparency with the Chinese government … we think lives could have been saved, we could have controlled it," Thompson said.[29]

The belief that China had covered up the initial SARS outbreak and allowed the disease to erupt across the world hit at the heart of what China had been working towards in the two decades since deciding to open up to the world and modernize its society. China's message to the world, conveyed most clearly in its application to join the World Trade Organization (WTO), had been that it was becoming a transparent, open, modern country that was aware of its responsibilities to the world. All of the effort that had been put into painting this picture of a transparent, open, modern China that was ready to assume its place as one of the world's great powers was put at risk by the clumsy handling of SARS.

It was not merely a question of image. China's economic

modernization was being jeopardized as well. The creation of a transparent business and legal environment was essential if the foreign investment necessary for modernization was to keep pouring in. China had worked hard to create a more open business environment. If it were seen to be returning to its old habits of secrecy, then this might well make foreign businesses pause before investing in China.

As SARS began to spread to different parts of China, and as international criticism of the government's conduct grew, the new leadership of President Hu Jintao and Premier Wen Jiabao acted fast to repair the damage that had been done. Health Minister Zhang Wenkang, who had steadfastly maintained the line that SARS was under control and that there was no reason for the outside world to be concerned, was removed from office. Vice Premier Wu Yi, a straight talking protégé of former premier Zhu Rongji was put in charge of battling SARS, and quickly won the respect of the international community for her openness.

Then Premier Wen, who had been plunged into the crisis barely a month after taking office, went to Bangkok for a summit meeting with ASEAN leaders where he acknowledged the mistakes that had been made. "I came to attend this conference in the spirit of candid responsibility, trust and cooperation," he declared. Instead of soothing words about the disease being under control, the Chinese premier warned that the disease was in danger of spreading to new parts of the country. "The number of SARS cases in Beijing, Shanxi and Inner Mongolia is rising noticeably. The situation has not been brought fully under control, and there is the tendency of spreading to more provinces in China."[30]

Never had a Chinese leader spoken so candidly about his country's internal problems and the failings of the government before an international audience. Clearly, a decisive shift in attitude towards the handling of SARS and the need to cooperate with the rest of the world in an open manner had occurred at the highest levels of the Chinese leadership.

Wen's speech was a sign that the wall of secrecy in China had been breached, and the fight against SARS in China was now integrated with what was going on in the rest of the world. Chinese doctors and researchers were now part of the worldwide network of research labs, clinicians and epidemiologists working on SARS. Due to the new leadership's rapid action in creating an electronic reporting system through which provinces could report their daily SARS figures to the Central government to be passed on to the WHO, accurate daily figures for SARS cases were available from every country in the world. The contact tracing and infection control measures that China had put in place on the WHO's recommendation meant that it now became possible to think about controlling the spread of SARS in China.

By the end of April 2003, six months after SARS first showed its face to the world, the Chinese government was no longer part of the problem. It had become part of the solution for controlling SARS.

* * *

With China on board, controlling SARS became a matter of making sure that a few basic principles were followed: suspected SARS cases had to be detected and placed in isolation, anyone they had been in contact with needed to be traced and monitored for signs of the disease and doctors, nurses and hospital workers needed to stick to the highest standards of infection control. As national health systems in the worst SARS-affected countries put together the machinery to do this, the number of cases gradually began to decline. Potential SARS patients were detected early, so they had less chance to spread the disease, and their families and friends were monitored or quarantined. By July 5, less than four months after the world was alerted to the presence of a new disease, the WHO was able to declare that the current epidemic had been contained. Taiwan, the last place where the disease had been spreading locally, had not reported a new case for 20 days, indicating that the chain of transmission had been stopped.

But at the WHO, beneath the exhaustion and the nervous tension, there was little feeling of triumph. There was no punching of the air, no champagne corks popping. The battle had been long and weary, but everyone knew the enemy had only been vanquished temporarily. The SARS virus was still present in nature, and it would probably be only a matter of time before it reappeared among humans. Gro Harlem Brundtland, in her last few weeks of office before stepping down as Director-General, marked the occasion with a sombre warning: "This is not the time to relax our vigilance. The world must remain on high alert for cases of SARS."[31]

There was, however, some reason for quiet satisfaction. The early warnings that David Heymann and his team had sounded had helped contain the disease. After the March 12 alert, although SARS had been reported in 30 countries, it did not spread locally in these countries. The case definition and the warnings issued by the WHO helped doctors and public health authorities to isolate suspected SARS patients and ensure that they did not spread the disease further. The only exception was Taiwan, where despite the health warnings, the disease took root and spread in the community. In China, Hong Kong, Vietnam, Singapore and Canada, SARS had already begun to spread before the WHO alert.

Fighting SARS had been a hard and stressful experience, the more so because the WHO has little real authority, and even less money. The organization has an annual budget of around US$800 million, an amount less than the budget of the average US hospital, as Ilona Kickbusch of Yale University's School of Public Health has pointed out[32]. To fund the bulk of its activities, the WHO runs around looking for donations from its member countries as well as wealthy foundations and charities.

When real action is needed, the financial constraints within which the WHO operates are compounded by its lack of political authority. When SARS broke out, the WHO did not have the authority to compel any of its member countries to either provide it with information, or to cooperate in any way. The WHO has a set of antiquated regulations that require countries to report only three diseases: cholera, plague and yellow fever. The legal requirement to notify the WHO of outbreaks of these diseases was laid down more than 40 years ago in the WHO's International Health Regulations, at a time when cholera, plague and yellow fever were thought to be the greatest threat to global public health.

The array of new infectious diseases that have cropped up since then have created the urgent need for a revision of these regulations that will give the WHO greater authority to ask for information from its members. In the absence of such authority, it was not merely China from which the WHO was finding it difficult to get information. During the SARS outbreak, the WHO also had problems getting data out of the US, like China, a country that is often uncomfortable in dealing with international organizations. Details of how the disease was spreading in the US were difficult to come by, and complicated by the fact that the CDC in Atlanta, the primary US disease-fighting agency, adopted its own case definition of SARS that varied slightly from the WHO's definition. Canada did the same, making it hard to tally figures for suspected and probable SARS cases globally.

Coming when it did, SARS allowed Brundtland to push WHO members to give the organization greater powers to investigate outbreaks and compel countries to release information. The WHO's decision-making body, the World Health Assembly, brings health ministers from all 181 member countries to Geneva every May to plan the organization's future work. In May 2003, the health ministers met at the height of the SARS crisis, and Brundtland used the opportunity to win their approval for a more activist role for the WHO.

The International Health Regulations, with their outdated list of diseases to be reported, were already in the process of being updated. But as is typical of decision making at the WHO, this was not expected to happen until 2005. Brundtland pushed for an earlier decision by the Health Assembly that would endorse a more activist role for the WHO and give it greater authority in dealing with governments and getting information out of countries.

The resolution, though conservatively worded to give individual countries as much leeway as possible, gave the WHO the power to alert the world if it felt that a public health threat existed in a particular country. It also allowed the WHO to take into account information gathered from credible non-official sources, not merely official sources, and gave guarded approval to the idea that the WHO could send teams to affected areas for on the spot studies. "This allows, within a country, for WHO to do what needs to be done to help the rest of the world," Brundtland said after the measures had been approved.[33]

The US, which is wary about giving international organizations too much authority, tried initially to block the proposal, worried that the international activities of its own CDC would come under question if the WHO received broader powers. "We understand the principle behind wanting to give the WHO more authority to take action. At the same time, we don't want in any way to crimp, impinge or limit the ability of the CDC to take action as well," a US government spokesman told *The Washington Post* at the time. But with the rest of the WHO's member states behind the move, the US too decided to back the resolution. It was clear to everyone that in an era in which diseases could spread so easily across the world, only a global organization would be able to fight them.

5

THE VIRUS HUNT

ON the morning of March 15, 2003, Chan Kwok-hung, a senior researcher at Hong Kong University, noticed a few clumpy patches in the normally even layer of cells growing on the sides of his test tubes. This seemingly mundane event, the death of a few cells in a test tube, was what the world of medicine had been waiting for. The SARS virus was showing itself for the first time in a laboratory, where it could be studied and analyzed.

At that point in mid-March, nothing seemed more important than trying to find the cause of SARS and stopping its spread. Once the virus was found, it would be possible to develop diagnostic tests to detect SARS patients and segregate them before they spread the disease. Identifying the agent responsible for SARS was also crucial to developing a vaccine and drugs for a disease that did not seem to respond to any of the existing antiviral drugs.

When SARS erupted in Hong Kong in early March, a small team of researchers at the Hong Kong University Faculty of Medicine found themselves propelled to the forefront of the global effort to identify the cause of the disease. Their medical colleagues were falling ill all around them, their city was paralyzed by fear and it was up to them to discover what was behind this epidemic.

This was a role for which they had been preparing. Hong Kong is one of the world's great trading cities, the place where China and the rest of the world meet to do business. It has also been the gateway through which diseases and epidemics originating on the vast Chinese mainland have passed to the outside world. In 1898, a plague epidemic that had originated in Yunnan province in southwest China some years earlier reached Hong Kong. From Hong Kong, it was carried to the rest of the world by trading vessels. In 1957 and in 1968, Hong Kong was the gateway through which lethal influenza viruses originating in southern China were exported to the outside world.[1] In 1997, a new bird flu virus erupted in Hong Kong and a possible pandemic was averted only after the Hong Kong government ordered the slaughter of all the chickens in the territory.[2]

If Hong Kong has been a gateway for disease, it has also worked to become a sentinel against disease, developing expertise in the early detection of epidemics. At the time of the SARS outbreak, much of this expertise was concentrated in the Microbiology Department at Hong Kong University, where the department head, K Y Yuen, had put together a team of scientists specializing in different disease-causing pathogens. The specialist in viral diseases was Malik Peiris, an Oxford educated scientist who would lead the efforts to discover the SARS virus.

Peiris has a reserved exterior that conceals both a lively sense of humour and a rigorous, analytical mind. Both these qualities were to serve him well during the outbreak. Peiris began his career in Sri Lanka investigating the spread of Japanese encephalitis in the early 1980s, but had focused his attention on influenza since arriving in Hong Kong in 1997 and was part of a Hong Kong University team that had built up an impressive pool of knowledge on human and avian flu viruses. Other team members included Guan Yi, an avian flu expert who would play a key role in researching the animal origins of the SARS virus.

Peiris and his team had begun to investigate the outbreak in southern China in early February, when rumours of a strange disease in Guangzhou reached Hong Kong. They knew that finding out what was happening in southern China required much more than scientific expertise. It required contacts in China. As Hong Kong researchers, Peiris and his team had absolutely no access to patients or to samples. They were like criminal investigators who were not allowed anywhere near the scene of the crime.

While goods, people and services flow smoothly across the boundary separating Hong Kong from Guangdong province, there are few official contacts between the Hong Kong government and the Guangdong provincial authorities. Hong Kong's special status as an autonomous region of China has meant that all official communication between Hong Kong and the rest of China is routed through the Central government in Beijing.

Anywhere else in the world, if a disease was raging in a neighbouring city, the obvious thing would be to pick up the phone and talk to the local health authorities to find out what was going on. For Hong Kong that was not possible. All formal communication had to go through the Central government in Beijing, a slow and tedious process.

At an informal level though, contacts between institutions on either side of the border have increased in the years since Hong Kong's return to China. Universities in Hong Kong have begun to collaborate with institutions on the mainland, and informal networks of researchers have also developed. These informal relationships played a crucial role in helping to breach the wall of official silence on SARS in China.

The Hong Kong University team was fortunate in that two of its members, Guan Yi and Zhen Bojian, were originally from mainland China, and had good contacts there. On February 12, both embarked on what amounted to a guerrilla mission to bring back samples from the mainland. Through the Institute of Respiratory Diseases in Guangzhou, they managed to bring back around 20 samples from SARS patients to Hong Kong. Officially, this was described as an "academic exchange" in order to get around Chinese laws.

This was a historic first opportunity for researchers outside of mainland China to crack the mystery of this new disease. The samples were taken to the Hong Kong University laboratory at Queen Mary Hospital, where Peiris and his team set to work.

The evidence at the time seemed to point to a mutant flu virus as the most plausible cause for the outbreak in Guangdong. Avian influenza, or bird flu, had been on the minds of epidemiologists since 1997, when a flu virus that normally infects only chickens and other birds jumped to humans. Unlike the normal flu virus, this avian virus, known as H5N1, proved to be particularly lethal to humans, killing 6 of the 18 people who contracted it. In February 2003, the avian virus reappeared in the human population, killing a 33-year-old Hong Kong man who had travelled to China during the Chinese New Year. His 9-year-old son was also infected by the virus, but recovered. These were the first cases of H5N1 since 1997, and the World Health Organization (WHO) went on alert for a possible flu pandemic.

Against this background, the outbreak of a mysterious respiratory disease in Guangdong seemed like another sign that a new flu virus was on the loose. So when the samples from China arrived in Hong Kong, the first step was to check whether they contained the H5N1 influenza virus.

To detect viruses, bacteria and other micro-organisms, microbiologists rely on a mixture of ancient and modern techniques. The giants of 19th century microbiology, Louis Pasteur and Robert Koch, discovered disease-causing agents by learning how to grow them in laboratories and observing them under a microscope. Cultivating a disease-causing organism in the laboratory and then seeing what it looks like under a microscope is still the gold standard of microbiological discovery. But this process is slow, and results are difficult to come by if the organism under investigation is difficult to cultivate in the laboratory. This is particularly true in the case of viruses. Unlike bacteria, which grow in any medium where the right nutrients are available, viruses can only reproduce in living cells. The only way to grow viruses in the laboratory is by culturing them in living cells in test tubes, or by injecting them into laboratory animals.

The development of serological tests in recent decades has given researchers a much quicker method of detecting micro-organisms. These are rapid laboratory tests that use the antibodies the human immune system produces when it is exposed to a disease-causing pathogen. These antibodies are specific to the organism they are meant to fight, and the presence of an antibody is a clear indication of infection by that agent. Serological tests either directly detect the presence of antibodies to a disease-causing agent in a patient's serum, or use antibodies to detect the presence of the agent itself. Serological tests such as radioimmunoassay (RIA) and enzyme-linked immunosorbent assay (ELISA) can detect the tiniest traces of either a disease-causing pathogen or antibodies to it in serum and other biological samples.

Advances in molecular biology have added another tool to the microbiologist's arsenal known as PCR, or polymerase chain reaction. Using PCR, researchers need only a tiny sliver of viral DNA or RNA to recreate large segments of the viral genome. They can then identify the virus based on its genetic structure.

Peiris first had the samples from China tested serologically for flu viruses as well as other respiratory viruses. None tested positive for H5N1 influenza. Some did show evidence of infection by a variety of common respiratory viruses, including an adenovirus, a human metapneumovirus and a normal human flu virus. But there was no trace of any pathogen that could cause a form of pneumonia as severe as that in Guangdong.

So the Hong Kong University team went back to basic principles and tried to grow any virus that might be present in the samples in cell cultures in test tubes. Since their main suspect was an influenza virus, the researchers used cell lines in which influenza viruses as well as other respiratory viruses grow. After more than a week of watching and waiting, nothing had happened, so the samples were put aside.

This was a fateful decision. Because at least one of the samples did in fact contain the SARS virus. But the virus did not grow in any of the cell lines that the Hong Kong University lab was using at the time. It was only a month later, after they had learned which cells lines the virus grew in, that researchers would come back to these early samples and find traces of the SARS virus.

Had the virus been teased out of these specimens at this stage, the world would have been alerted several weeks earlier, and the spread of the new disease might have been contained. K Y Yuen, the head of the Department of Microbiology at Hong Kong University who oversaw the research team, felt the burden of this missed opportunity: "We were thinking of H5N1 and used cell lines specific to this virus. So we failed to culture the real SARS virus. It was a missed opportunity, and we have to be honest about it."[3]

In retrospect, it would have taken a stroke of extraordinary luck to have unearthed the SARS virus at that stage in early February. SARS had not even been identified as a new disease, and Peiris and his team were not really looking for an unknown virus. From the little that was known in the outside world about the disease in Guangdong, it seemed to be either a flu or a viral pneumonia of some kind.

"It was not at all clear at that stage that we were looking at something unknown," Peiris recalled. "The only unusual thing about the disease, was that health care workers seemed to get affected disproportionately. But a particularly severe influenza could conceivably have produced this same effect. Our first concern was eliminate all the common or garden viruses."[4]

At the best of times, finding a new virus requires an element of luck. Even though microbiologists have a wide array of sophisticated serological and molecular tests to identify viruses and other micro-organisms in tissue and serum samples, these tests are suited to detecting known viruses. Finding a new virus requires going back to the oldest of microbiological techniques: growing the virus either in live laboratory animals or in cell cultures in test tubes. The SARS virus is not particularly easy to grow in cell culture, and it failed to grow in any of the cell lines that were used for these early samples.

Until the second week of March, the search for the new virus was largely an academic exercise to identify a disease that was happening somewhere else. On March 12, all of that changed. The disease erupted outside China, exploding almost simultaneously in Hong Kong, Singapore, Hanoi and Toronto. In Hong Kong, panic spread through the health system, and Peiris and his team found themselves grappling with the virus in their midst.

"The pressure was enormous," recalled John Nicholls, a pathologist at the University who had been roped in by Peiris to join the small team searching for the SARS virus. "After the Prince of Wales outbreak and the outbreak in Hanoi, it was really all systems go. People were terrified, businesses were getting affected. We just had to find out what it was."[5]

Samples poured into the laboratory. In the early stages, Peiris was not sure that the samples he was getting were actually from SARS patients. The WHO's initial definition of the disease was broad, and in Hong Kong, it embraced virtually anyone with a severe pneumonia that did not respond to antibiotics. The team was battling two unknowns at the same time: looking for an unknown disease in samples from patients they were not even sure had the disease.

There was one sample they were fairly sure about though. On March 4, they received a lung biopsy sample from Chan Ying-pui, the brother-in-law of Liu Jianlun, the professor from Guangzhou who had brought the disease to Hong Kong. Chan had also fallen ill with what was clearly SARS. The biopsy had been taken while he was still alive, increasing the chance that the virus causing the disease was still present in the tissue.

The challenge now was to tease the virus out of the tissue. The researchers ground up the lung tissue and injected it into test tubes with different cell lines. If they were lucky, the virus would infect these cells and multiply in the test tubes, making it easy to detect and identify.

Persuading a virus to grow in a cell culture in test tubes is not easy. Viruses are finicky about which cells they will infect, and the virologist must have a combination of skill, experience and luck to isolate a difficult virus. Patience is another essential quality. Viruses can take two weeks or more to infect cells in a culture. Waiting for a virus to show itself is largely a matter of leaving test tubes in incubators warmed to body temperature, and examining them every day under a microscope for evidence of infection.

The Hong Kong University team used a variety of cell lines that were known to be useful in growing respiratory viruses. But after more than a week, there was little sign of activity in any of the cell cultures. As frustration grew, the virologists decided to add a cell line of fetal kidney cells from rhesus monkeys to see whether this would yield results. This was a cell line that the Hong Kong University team rarely used, but which had proved useful in growing another respiratory virus, the human metapneumovirus. It proved to be an inspired choice.

Material from the lung biopsy was introduced into the new cell culture on March 13. It was in this new culture that two days later, on March 15, Chan Kwok-hung, the Hong Kong University researcher, noticed something unusual had happened. The cells appeared to be dying. But was it due to the SARS virus, or to some other infection? "I was excited," Chan recalled. "But I was worried whether this was really the SARS virus causing it, or whether it was some kind of secondary infection in the test tubes."[6]

Being a cautious man, Chan said nothing to his boss Malik Peiris, but decided to wait out the weekend and see whether the test tubes showed more definite signs of cell death. The following Monday, Peiris himself noticed the clustering of cells, and talked it over with Chan. Chan was still sceptical: there had been little change over the weekend, and if the SARS virus was in fact at work, it appeared to be working very slowly.

The two decided to re-inject the fluid into new test tubes with fresh cells to avoid the possibility that the old cells were dying of contamination. Once again, the cells started dying off, this time at a much faster rate. Clearly, this was not due to contamination. A virus was multiplying and killing the cells in the test tubes.

Peiris and his team had succeeded in growing a virus that had been present in a SARS patient. But they still had to establish that the virus they had isolated was in fact the virus that caused SARS and not an incidental infection. Humans can be infected with a number of different viruses at the same time and it was crucial to determine whether this particular virus was the causal agent for SARS.

More than a century ago, the great German microbiologist Robert Koch set out a series of steps for determining the causative agent for a disease. These postulates have been modified over time, but the scientific logic behind them is enduring. Koch stated that the disease-causing agent had to be isolated in a culture, after which it had to be demonstrated that this agent was in fact present in anyone with the disease.

Peiris and his team had accomplished the first step: isolating a possible causative agent for SARS. The next step was to see whether this virus was in fact present in other SARS cases. This was done through a serological test. Serum from SARS patients would contain antibodies to the SARS virus. If those antibodies reacted with the virus that they had isolated, then the virus was definitely the agent causing the disease. On March 18 and 19, the Hong Kong University team tested their virus against blood serum samples from patients at different stages of the disease, from early onset to the late stages. The viral material in the test tubes was extracted and put onto slides. Then, serum from SARS patients was introduced into the material on the slides. To the gratification of the researchers, the antibodies in the blood samples reacted to the virus on the slides. Not only did the blood serum react, the strength of the reaction increased in serum samples taken later in the course of the disease. This rising antibody response indicated a strong association between the virus they had isolated and the disease. Peiris was now increasingly confident that he had the virus in his grasp. "We had the virus growing well, it was reacting in the expected way to early and late serum samples. We were quite sure this was the virus causing SARS."[7]

The virus was now growing in test tubes where it could be studied and analyzed. But the Hong Kong University team was not quite ready to go public. For one thing, researchers were not quite sure what kind of virus it was. This would require visual identification using an electron microscope, as well as an analysis of its genetic structure using PCR. John Nicholls, the pathologist, set to work trying to identify the virus visually, while a young researcher, Leo Poon, began extracting sequences of the virus' genetic structure for examination.

Peiris is a cautious scientist, slow to jump to conclusions unless he is absolutely sure about them. So even before announcing his preliminary findings to fellow scientists in the global network of research labs that the WHO had organized to search for the SARS virus, he decided to test the virus independently in a "blind test" against serum samples from patients with and without SARS.

On March 21, the Hong Kong government's virology lab organized the test by providing six samples, three from SARS patients, and three from people without SARS. The researchers did not know which samples came from SARS patients and which did not, and had to distinguish between the two groups using the virus they had isolated. Once again, the antibodies in the serum from the three SARS patients reacted to the virus, while the other samples did not react at all.

That afternoon, John Nicholls took his first look at the new virus through an electron microscope. The tiny viral particles surrounded by little dots were unlike anything he had seen before. As he flipped through a book of electron microscope pictures of viruses, Nicholls realized that the halo of dots surrounding the virus was strongly suggestive of a coronavirus. This was a surprise, as coronaviruses had been nowhere on the suspect list when the hunt for the SARS virus began. Coronaviruses, so named because of their distinctive crown-like ring of proteins, cause respiratory and enteric infections in a wide range of animals, including cattle, pigs, rodents and chickens, and their study is largely the province of virologists specializing in animal viruses. The only two kinds of coronavirus known to infect humans cause colds and

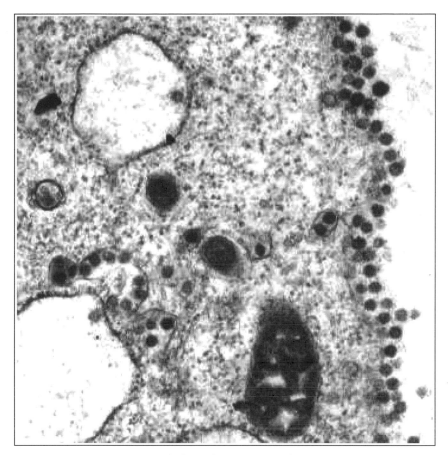

Coronavirus (Courtesy J.W.Nicholls and J.S.M. Peiris, The University of Hong Kong).

mild respiratory illnesses. No coronavirus had ever been known to cause a disease as serious as SARS in humans.

Two days later, more detailed pictures from the Hong Kong government virology lab confirmed Nicholl's initial belief that this was a coronavirus. Genetic analysis also showed fragments of genetic material that were distinctive to the coronavirus family, though there were parts of the virus' genome that seemed different from all other known coronaviruses.

At the end of the day on March 21, the Hong Kong University team were sure they had isolated the virus causing SARS: the testing against serum samples had shown a clear association between the virus they had found and antibodies in SARS patients. Electron microscope pictures had revealed a virus that might be a coronavirus.

Peiris felt confident enough of these results to notify his colleagues. That evening, he emailed Klaus Stohr, the scientist coordinating the WHO's global efforts to identify the SARS virus, to let him know that the Hong Kong team had found the pathogen causing SARS.

* * *

As described in Chapter 4, the WHO had brought together a global network of research institutions to find the SARS virus on March 17, the same day that Peiris and his team saw signs of viral activity in their test tubes. Peiris was part of the WHO network but felt his findings were too premature to mention at this time. All he had was evidence of viral activity in test tubes in his lab. He had done none of the tests that would indicate that the virus that had been isolated was in fact the SARS virus.

On the following two days, March 18 and 19, while Peiris was still setting up various confirmatory tests, several laboratories around the world announced that they had found traces of a virus that was a possible causative agent for SARS. The virus these researchers had isolated, however, was not a coronavirus, but a type of paramyxovirus, a viral family that includes the measles and mumps viruses.

In Germany, a group of scientists from the Bernard Nocht Institute in Hamburg and the Institute for Medical Virology at Goethe University in Frankfurt reported that they had seen viral particles that resembled the paramyxovirus under an electron microscope. A day later, they announced they had also found evidence of the virus in a blood sample from a SARS patient, making it more likely that this was the causative agent.[8]

Fifteen miles away from Hong Kong University, the research team at the Chinese University of Hong Kong also announced that it had found a virus that was a member of the paramyxovirus family, a human metapneumovirus, in samples from hospital workers who had contracted SARS at the Prince of Wales Hospital. A news release by Chinese University said that researchers had "identified the virus that caused the recent outbreak" as a member of the paramyxovirus family.[9] On the same day, the Pathology Department at the Singapore General Hospital and Singapore's Defence Medical Research Institute identified a paramyxovirus as the most likely cause for SARS. "Preliminary investigations by the Pathology Department at the Singapore General Hospital and the Defence Medical Research Institute have identified the likely infective agent to belong to the paramyxovirus family," a Ministry of Health news release said.[10] Almost simultaneously, Canadian scientists at the National Microbiology Laboratory in Winnipeg announced they had found evidence of the human metapneumovirus in six of the eight samples they were analyzing.[11]

Buffeted by these claims coming in from all over the world that a paramyxovirus was the causative agent for SARS, Peiris was sure of two things: first, that he had the real SARS virus in his hands, and second, that whatever type of virus it was, it was not a paramyxovirus or a human metapneumovirus. "We had tested the virus by PCR to see if it was a paramyxovirus, and it was not," he recalled.[12]

All the other laboratories appeared to be basing their findings on having seen paramyxovirus-like particles under an electron microscope, or on having found genetic traces of the virus in patients' samples. But none of them had grown the virus from patients' samples and tested it against serum from known SARS patients to see whether what they had was the SARS virus. Without taking this step, they were in the position of policemen who had found fingerprints at the scene of a crime, but had no evidence that these were the fingerprints of the criminal.

At research laboratories all over the world though, the paramyxovirus became the prime suspect, and the WHO network turned its attention to confirming whether a paramyxovirus was the causal agent for SARS. At the time, a paramyxovirus seemed a plausible candidate. Two new members of this family had emerged recently to cause disease in humans: the Nipah virus in Malaysia, which caused an encephalitis-like disease, and the related Hendra virus in Australia. Given the wide range of animals and reptiles that carry paramyxoviruses, from horses in North America to tree shrews in Thailand, it was not difficult to conceive that a new paramyxovirus had passed from animals to humans and caused SARS.

On March 21, Klaus Stohr, the coordinator for the WHO global research network, announced that "more and more laboratories were finding paramyxovirus," adding that it seemed to be a virus that was unlike any of the known members of this family. David Heymann, the WHO Executive Director heading its anti-SARS effort, told a news conference that morning that "we are now closer to reality that this Paramyxoviridae virus has caused this."[13]

Later in the day, Peiris' email arrived at the WHO announcing that his team had isolated a virus and confirming that it was the causal agent for SARS. The breakthrough caused excitement at the WHO headquarters, and Stohr put out a press release describing it as a "real ray of sunshine." The assumption in Geneva, however, was that this was probably a new kind of paramyxovirus. "The infectious agent resembles the morphology of a paramyxovirus. Scientists cannot, however be certain about the identity of the virus, which may indeed be a new paramyxovirus, or another a virus with a similar morphology," the WHO press release said.[14]

This was clearly a time of some confusion. But Peiris' email served to turn the attention of the WHO network away from the paramyxovirus to the real causative agent, the coronavirus. In an article in *Lancet* that looked back on this period, Klaus Stohr described the findings from Hong Kong as "a turning point in the search for the causative agent."[15] This moment was significant for a number of reasons. First, the Hong Kong team had now managed to isolate the SARS virus from two patients. In addition to the samples from Chan Ying-pui, tissue from a woman who had been infected on a visit to Guangzhou also contained the virus, strengthening the credibility of the findings. Second, the team had done a blind test with the virus against serum from SARS patients as well as those without SARS, and found that only serum from SARS patients contained antibodies to the virus. The levels of antibodies to the virus also increased in the serum as the disease progressed, indicating a clear association between the virus and the disease. And finally, electron microscope pictures had revealed the presence of the virus in infected cells.

After the announcement from Hong Kong, other laboratories began to find the coronavirus. On March 21, the National Influenza Centre at Erasmus University in Rotterdam and the Institute for Medical Virology at Goethe University in Frankfurt each announced that they had isolated a virus, but neither had tested it to determine whether this was the virus causing SARS. Three days later, both laboratories confirmed that the new virus was in fact a coronavirus.

The Hong Kong University findings were boosted the next day by the Centers for Disease Control and Prevention (CDC) in Atlanta, the largest and best resourced disease-fighting organization in the world. The CDC informed the WHO network that it had isolated a virus and identified it as a coronavirus based on electron microscope pictures, which were put up on the WHO's secure website. The Hong Kong government virology lab also sent the WHO electron microscope photographs clearly indicating a coronavirus on the same day.[16]

But there were still contradictory results coming in from some of the laboratories, particularly in Canada, where traces of the human metapneumovirus were found in the first few samples. Frank Plummer, the head of Canada's National Microbiology Laboratory, remained sceptical that the coronavirus was the causative agent for SARS. In an interview with *Science* magazine in April, Plummer said that only 50 percent of Canadian patients who met the case definition for SARS tested positive for the coronavirus. Plummer's lab was also finding only very small amounts of virus in the samples that did test positive. "The coronavirus is definitely around in the environment, it's definitely circulating, but the relationship with SARS, based on our data appears to be fairly weak," he said. "The chances of having SARS if you have this virus are increased by about a factor of two — compared with if you don't." Plummer was also dubious about the human metapneumovirus as a causal agent for SARS. "We find the metapneumovirus in a few patients, but there's not really a correlation," he said.[17]

With some laboratories reporting findings of the paramyxovirus, researchers also looked at the possibility that both viruses were required to cause the disease. As Klaus Stohr suggested, perhaps "these two pathogens have come together to cause this very severe outbreak ... what we could hypothesize is that this coronavirus destroys, or at least diminishes the immunity in the patient so that the second virus has practically an open door to go in and sicken the patient beyond what the virus would do normally."[18]

A disease with two causal agents would be highly unusual, but not impossible. To test the hypothesis that SARS had two causal agents, an experiment with macaque monkeys was set up at Erasmus University in Rotterdam by Albert Osterhaus, one of the scientists in the WHO laboratory network. One group of monkeys was infected with the coronavirus, another group was infected with the human metapneumovirus and a third group was infected with both viruses. Osterhaus described what happened:

> The animals infected with the coronavirus alone developed full blown disease. They developed SARS, they developed clinical symptoms, and they also developed the pathological lesions that are identical to what we have seen in persons who died of SARS. The animals with the human metapneumovirus developed only a mild rhinitis, they had very mild symptoms, and definitely not the typical SARS pattern. The third group of animals, first infected with the coronavirus, and then super infected with the metapneumovirus did not develop more serious disease.[19]

The conclusion was that the coronavirus was the causal agent for SARS, and that it was both a necessary as well as a sufficient cause for SARS. Even if other pathogens like the human metapneumovirus were associated with SARS, Osterhaus' experiments showed that the coronavirus alone was sufficient to cause SARS. The coronavirus was also necessary to cause SARS: without it, the disease would not develop.

This conclusion was backed by another study using data from 463 SARS patients from all parts of the world except the US and Canada, which showed that the coronavirus was present in 75 percent of cases, while only 12 percent of cases were co-infected with the human metapneumovirus.[20]

These experiments confirmed the original Hong Kong University findings, and brought to a close a remarkable global scientific effort. It had taken just over a month from the time the new disease erupted outside of China in the second week of March 2003 to identify its cause conclusively. This was astonishingly fast compared to the time it has taken to identify the causes of other new diseases that have emerged in the last few decades. It took more than two years for scientists to discover the AIDS virus. The bacteria that causes Legionnaires disease took five months to track down.

Part of the reason it was possible to work this quickly was the collaboration between some of the world's foremost microbiologists, who exchanged information and ideas through a daily teleconference. This helped researchers concentrate on promising lines of enquiry, and speeded up the process by which findings could be confirmed or rejected.

The normal competition between scientists and research institutes did not, however, disappear overnight. SARS was the first new infectious disease to cause a global health scare since the emergence of AIDS nearly 20 years earlier. The opportunity to detect a new virus that has caused a global health scare comes rarely to most scientists. And when it does come along, there is no scientist who does not want to be the first to find it. It is based on discoveries like this that scientific reputations are built.

And so there was heartburn not only in Hong Kong, but elsewhere as well, that much of the credit for uncovering the SARS virus appeared to have gone to the CDC. On March 24, the CDC issued a news release and held a press conference in Atlanta announcing that a new coronavirus was the "leading hypothesis" for the cause of SARS. The news release, as well as the press conference by the CDC Director, Julie Gerberding, mentioned the work of the WHO collaborative network, but the underlying message was that the CDC had made the big breakthrough and isolated the virus first.[21]

WHO officials knew the role that Peiris and his team had played in isolating the virus and tried to set the record straight several times during various press conferences. "Just so you are clear, the virus was first found in Hong Kong, first identified in Hong Kong. And then it was identified in the CDC. And now it has been identified by all the other laboratories," David Heymann, the WHO Executive Director, told the Geneva press corps.[22]

In the world of science, it is not media announcements, but results published in professional journals that are the true index of achievement. And here Peiris and his colleagues got their recognition. Their paper published in the online edition of *Lancet* on April 8 was the first scientific paper describing the new coronavirus as the causal agent for SARS.[23] A paper by the CDC group describing its findings was published two days later in the *New England Journal of Medicine*, as was a paper by the group of European scientists in Germany and the Netherlands.[24] Whether by intention or by chance, the two-day gap in publication between the Hong Kong paper and the two other papers reflected the gap by which the Hong Kong team had pipped other research teams to the post.

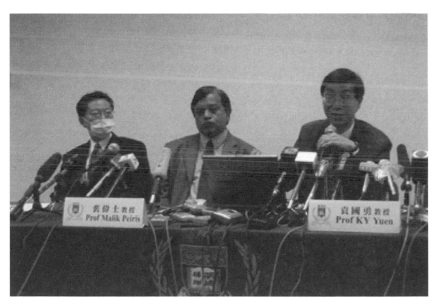

Malik Peiris (center), K.Y. Yuen (right), head of the Department of Microbiology, and S.K. Lam (left, Dean of the Medical Faculty at the University of Hong Kong, at a press conference on SARS.

For the Hong Kong University team, finding the SARS virus was a vindication of the traditional methods of science: careful conclusions drawn from meticulously conducted experiments. The conflicting findings of different labs also showed that despite the technological advances of the past few decades, detecting micro-organisms, particularly new ones, is not easy. Molecular techniques such as PCR that can detect a virus through its genes have revolutionized the way microbiologists work, but these techniques are not infallible.

In the end, it was the time-tested techniques pioneered by Pasteur and Koch that led to the identification of the SARS virus: isolating the infectious agent by culturing it in the laboratory, and then proving that the virus or bacteria that has been isolated is in fact the agent responsible for the disease by using it to cause fresh infection in living organisms.

Malik Peiris is a virologist who believes in the value of the traditional methods of science. Reminiscing on a Saturday morning in June in his small office overflowing with books, papers and files, he pointed out with some satisfaction that the tried and trusted methods were the ones that had worked in the end. "There's an important virological lesson here," he mused. "You have all these new fangled approaches — gene sequencing, PCR and so on. But the real breakthrough came from old fashioned virology — growing the thing, and then seeing it."[25]

Peiris led a small team that produced results ahead of laboratories many times larger than his own. He summed up the key to scientific success in the following way: "Keep your feet on the ground, don't get carried away, be cautious, and nail things down thoroughly before coming to conclusions."[26]

There was clearly an element of good fortune involved as well: the Hong Kong team had access to samples and were in the thick of the epidemic, the best place for an investigator to be. But good fortune does not explain everything. As Louis Pasteur put it, fortune only favours the prepared mind.

* * *

As SARS raged through southern China in February and March, Chinese scientists and researchers were also busy trying to isolate the agent that was causing the disease. They had one advantage over researchers elsewhere: access to a large number of samples well before the disease had actually been recognized in the outside world. But they had a huge handicap as well: institutional and political constraints that shut some of the country's best researchers out of the race to identify the virus.

When the disease broke out in Guangdong in February 2003, researchers in the province as well as at the national Centre for Diseases Control and Prevention (CDC) in Beijing, the body in charge of handling epidemics, began testing samples from patients. On February 18, there appeared to be an early breakthrough when the head of the CDC, Li Liming, announced that his researchers had isolated the chlamydia bacteria from SARS samples, and that this was the possible causative agent for the disease.[27]

The announcement was greeted with some scepticism. It was quite possible that signs of chlamydia had been found in the samples. One member of the chlamydia family, *C. pneumoniae*, was known to cause community-acquired pneumonia. But demonstrating the presence of the bacteria in samples was not the same as proving that it was the agent causing the disease. And it was unlikely that chlamydia was responsible for a disease as severe as the illness that had been seen in Guangzhou. Pneumonia caused by chlamydia is easily treatable with antibiotics. Physicians in Guangzhou who had been battling the disease knew that antibiotics were useless, and so chlamydia and other bacterial agents were unlikely to be the cause. Zhong Nanshan, the doctor who spearheaded the battle against SARS in Guangdong, was a member of the Chinese Academy of Sciences and high enough in the scientific hierarchy to challenge these findings, and to refuse to follow the CDC's recommendation that antibiotics be used to treat the disease. At a meeting on February 20, Zhong and other doctors from Guangdong disagreed with the CDC, and said that they would continue to treat the disease as if it were a viral disease. "We thought their [the CDC's] conclusion was false. We had been using antibiotics from early February, but found they did not have any effect ... We insisted on treating the disease according to our own investigations," he said in an interview on the Chinese CCTV television network in June. The media in Guangdong and elsewhere was forbidden from reporting on the dispute over the cause of SARS, and the CDC's theory remained unchallenged in public.

But the fact that the national CDC, the body at the apex of China's disease-fighting infrastructure, had announced that chlamydia was the causal agent made it difficult for anyone else to challenge this finding publicly, despite private doubts. Once chlamydia as the causative agent for SARS became the official truth, no questioning of this theory or discussion of more plausible causes was possible. The fact that a senior microbiologist at the CDC, Hong Tao, had been responsible for identifying chlamydia made it even more difficult for other researchers to challenge this finding.

Chinese officials were reluctant to accept the idea that a newly discovered coronavirus was the causal agent for the disease. As late as April 4, when the rest of the world was working to learn more about the coronavirus, Chinese authorities were still announcing they had made a breakthrough in linking chlamydia to SARS. At a press conference on that day, Li Liming, the CDC Director, said "Chinese experts have successfully separated a chlamydia-like agent from the bodies of five SARS victims and the agent can be basically confirmed as the prime culprit of the disease." He acknowledged that the possibility that SARS was caused by a coronavirus could not be discounted, but maintained that he had evidence that chlamydia was the primary cause of the disease. "Undoubtedly Chinese experts are very likely to become the first to find the cause of the disease," he said.[28]

The magazine *Science* has reported that a team of Chinese researchers might actually have isolated the SARS virus as early as the end of February, but was reluctant to publicize its findings.[29] A team of researchers at the Academy of Military and Medical Sciences had obtained patient samples from the military hospital in Guangzhou on February 14, and cultured the virus by February 22. Two days later they took electron micrograph pictures of the new virus, which had the tell-tale coronavirus spikes. By the first week of March, the research team of Zhu Qingyu and Yang Ruifu found that their virus reacted with serum from SARS patients, indicating that they had in fact isolated the virus causing the disease.

The researchers told *Science* that they had not publicized their findings because they had not wanted to challenge the CDC findings. "It would not have been respectful," Yang Ruifu told the magazine. The researchers had only a limited amount of serum to validate their results, and were apparently not confident enough of these results to go public. "We all wanted to be sure. Dr Hong Tao [of the CDC] is very famous in China. We had to show respect," Yang told the magazine.

If the team had managed to isolate the SARS virus and publicize its results in early March, then the course of the SARS epidemic might have been different. Early identification of the virus would probably have speeded up the development of efficient diagnostic tests, which in turn would have enabled the early identification and hospitalization of SARS patients.

Other research institutions on the mainland were also handicapped by bureaucratic obstacles. At the Beijing Genomics Institute, China's top genetic research institute, researchers struggled to get hold of hold of viral samples for sequencing. Officially, only the CDC was authorized to obtain samples from SARS patients, and there was no way anyone else could get hold of samples. Yang Huanming, the Director of the Institute, revealed that beginning in February, their scientists had gone to Guangdong several times in an effort to get samples of the virus, but had been unsuccessful each time. "We had been hoping to make a contribution since we knew about it...we had been looking for original samples of the pathogen since February," Yang said.[30] On April 14, a day after Canadian researchers sequenced the SARS genome, the frustrated scientists managed to get samples from an as yet unnamed research institute using their personal contacts. Because the transaction was illegal, the researchers had to adopt cloak and dagger methods to get the samples. "We had to go there after 10 p.m. and before 7 a.m. We had to wear hats and masks for disguise when we met. It made us feel we were conducting spying activities," one researcher said.

Two days later the Institute finished sequencing four different isolates, an impressive rate of work that might have allowed researchers to be the first in the world to sequence the gene had they been given access to samples.

It was only after the political shake-up at the Ministry of Health toward the end of April, when Health Minister Zhang Wenkang and the Mayor of Beijing, Meng Xuenong, were dismissed, that the constraints on research on the SARS virus were removed. China's president, Hu Jintao, visited the Academy of Military and Medical Sciences and congratulated the scientists for the work they had done, lending official legitimacy to their work. Some of the obstacles to cooperation between researchers from different institutions were also removed after a national scientific task force on SARS was created.

*　*　*

Armed with boxes of bottles and swabs and carrying 10 000 Hong Kong dollars in his pockets, associate professor Guan Yi of Hong Kong University walked into the main animal market in Shenzhen, the Chinese border town that adjoins Hong Kong. It was an afternoon in early May, and as the main business of the day had been transacted during the morning, the market was quiet and trade was slow. Cages that were normally full of badgers, civets, racoons, rabbits, barking deer and a variety of other animals destined for cooking pots in restaurants and homes across the city, were nearly empty.

But there were still a few traders around, hoping to catch late customers. In their cages were palm civets, small, brown racoon-like creatures with white stripes down their muzzles and around their eyes, hog badgers with long snouts, beavers and rabbits. Guan Yi's mission was simple: to determine whether these creatures carried in them a coronavirus related to the SARS virus.

After the SARS virus had been identified in March, the search began to discover how it had emerged. Molecular biologists in laboratories around the world began deciphering its genetic code to look for clues. On April 12, the Michael Smith Genome Sciences Centre in British Columbia, Canada, announced that it had sequenced the entire genome of the SARS virus.[31]

Its genetic structure confirmed that the SARS virus was a coronavirus. Its genes were organized into a chain of nearly 30 000 nucleotides, molecules made up of RNA, sugar and phosphate. Different sections of the viral genome contained the instructions to create the proteins that make up the different parts of a virus: the spikes it uses to latch on to host cells; the capsid, or cover, that encloses the viral genes; the membrane that envelopes the virus; and the various enzymes the virus needs to hijack the cellular machinery and reproduce itself.

Viruses, like all forms of life on earth, carry the genetic instructions necessary for their reproduction in the form of nucleic acids. While more complex forms of life have their genes encoded as DNA, or deoxyribonucleic acid, the genetic information of a virus may be stored either as DNA or as RNA, ribonucleic acid. The SARS coronavirus, like other members of the coronavirus family, is an RNA virus. RNA is a less stable nucleic acid form than DNA. Most life forms use RNA only as a messenger to carry DNA instructions, and not for permanent storage of their genes. Because RNA is less stable, when an RNA virus reproduces, mistakes, or mutations, occur far more frequently than in DNA-based genomes. RNA averages one error, or mutation, for every 10 000 nucleotides copied. For DNA, this number can be as low as one error in every 10 million nucleotides. This rapid mutation is part of an RNA virus' survival mechanism: because it changes so rapidly, it is easier for the virus to evade the immune system of its host, and re-infect the host.

When a coronavirus finds a host cell with receptors into which its spikes will fit, it infects the cell and transfers its genetic material into the cell. It then hijacks the host cell's protein-building machinery to create copies of itself. Within a short period of infection, large numbers of new viruses are created, exploding out of the host cell to infect new cells.

As researchers painstakingly identified each of the tiny nucleotides that carried the codes for the SARS virus' spike, outer membrane, capsid and other essential proteins, they found distinct differences with all other known coronaviruses. Until the discovery of the SARS virus, coronaviruses had been divided into three broad families based on their genetic structure and the hosts they infected. Group one and group three coronaviruses infected mammals, while group two coronaviruses infected birds. The two coronaviruses known to infect humans and cause colds were in group one and group three. The SARS virus though, did not fit easily into any of these groups, and appeared to represent a new group of its own. As Marco Marra, the scientist who led the Canadian group that first sequenced the SARS virus, wrote, "This SARS virus is not more closely related to any of the three known classes of coronavirus and we propose that it defines a fourth class of coronavirus."[32]

By examining the genome of the SARS virus and comparing it with other coronaviruses, molecular epidemiologists hoped to solve the riddle of how this virus had originated. There were several possibilities, some far-fetched, others more plausible.

As happens when any new disease arises, conspiracy theorists quickly decided that this virus must have been created as a biological weapon in a military laboratory somewhere. Sergei Kolesnikov, a member of the Russian Academy of Medical Sciences, enjoyed a brief moment in the media spotlight when his comments that the SARS virus was a man-made synthesis of the measles and mumps virus were widely reported internationally.[33] Others speculated that the SARS virus had escaped from a Chinese biological weapons facility.[34] The British astronomer, Chandra Wickremasinghe of Cardiff University, who has long believed that many viruses and bacteria found on earth came from outer space, suggested in a letter to the *Lancet* that the SARS virus might have extra-terrestrial origins.[35]

As these far-fetched theories buzzed around internet chat rooms, researchers were also testing more plausible theories. One possibility was that the SARS virus was a mutated form of one of the two known human coronaviruses. But the genetic differences between the SARS virus and the other human coronaviruses were too significant to have made this feasible. The most likely explanation was that the SARS virus was not a newly evolved virus, but rather an animal coronavirus that had been living undiscovered in an animal host for perhaps thousands of years before passing to humans.

This had been the pattern with other newly emergent diseases such as AIDS and Ebola, which were caused by animal viruses that had jumped from their natural animal host to humans. The possibility that the SARS virus had animal origins was backed by data from Guangdong that showed that more than a third of the early cases in southern China were food handlers who could have come in contact with exotic meats. If this was the case, the virus could have passed to humans in the markets where exotic live animals were sold for both food and medicinal purposes in southern China.

This was what Guan Yi had come to Shenzhen to find out. Backed by researchers from the Shenzhen Centre for Diseases Control and Prevention and the local authorities, he negotiated with the traders: could he take blood samples and swabs from their animals? He would have to anesthetize them first, but this would not harm the animals, he assured traders. In the face of scepticism from traders who saw their produce being killed, Guan produced his trump card: he had 10 000 Hong Kong dollars, he declared, and would buy any animal that died or was harmed in any way in the sampling process.

Faced with this largesse, the doubts evaporated, and the researchers got to work, gingerly pulling reluctant animals out of their cages, carefully avoiding sharp claws and teeth, drawing blood samples and collecting nasal and faecal swabs. It was tough going, and by the end of the day, they had only managed to collect samples from nine animals. The next morning, there was a wider array of animals for sale: barking deer, racoon dogs and Chinese ferret badgers. At the end of two days, the researchers had managed to get 25 samples from a wide variety of animals, as well as blood samples from traders at the market.

The samples showed that four out of six of the palm civets tested carried a coronavirus that was 99.8 percent genetically identical to the human coronavirus. One of the racoon dogs carried the same virus as the civet cats, while one ferret badger had antibodies to the virus, indicating that it had been infected at some stage in its life. When the animal viruses were sequenced, they were found to have a short section of 29 nucleotides that was missing in the human virus. The absence of this section, perhaps through a random mutation, could have been what allowed the virus to transmit easily between humans.[36]

Forty percent of the animal traders whose blood was tested and 20 percent of those involved in slaughtering the animals had antibodies to the virus carried by the civet cats, indicating that the virus was passing between animals and humans. This indicated that a SARS-like coronavirus had been circulating among palm civets and other animals in markets in southern China as well as among market traders, apparently without causing disease.

A study by epidemiologists at the Guangdong Centre for Disease Control also provided evidence for the suggested link between animal trading and the SARS virus. When traders in three animal markets in Guangdong province were tested, 13.9 percent of them were found to have antibodies to SARS, even though none of them had contracted the disease. Those who traded in palm civets, wild boar and deer were found to be most likely to have antibodies to SARS.[37]

All of this pointed to the virus passing from animals to humans in the marketplaces of southern China. But it did not answer the crucial question of where the virus normally resided in nature, or indicate the path the virus had taken from its natural host to humans. While four civet cats at the market in Shenzhen were found to carry the coronavirus, there were subtle genetic differences in the virus they carried. This indicated they had been infected by some other animal in the wild, or on the farms where they were bred. In an article reporting their findings in the magazine *Science*, Guan Yi and his colleagues wrote, "It is conceivable that civets, raccoon-dogs and ferret badgers were all infected from yet another unknown animal source, which is in fact the true reservoir in nature ... these market animals may be intermediate hosts that increase the opportunity for transmission of infection to humans."[38] In other words, the markets, where different species of animals were caged in close proximity to each other, provided a venue for the virus to pass between animals and to jump from animals to humans. But the real source existed elsewhere.

While the virus may have been living in an animal host for centuries, researchers like Malik Peiris believe it has been circulating in the human population for some decades, causing small outbreaks of disease and gradually evolving and becoming better at transmitting between humans. Peiris bases this belief on the fact that the SARS virus, unlike most other new viruses that have recently emerged from the animal population, transmits easily between humans. When a virus first crosses from animals to humans, it does not have the ability to transmit readily from human to human. It takes a while for the virus to adapt to the requirements of its new human host. The SARS virus was already fairly well adapted to humans.[39]

Another hypothesis is that the SARS virus is the result of an avian coronavirus and a mammalian coronavirus exchanging genes to create a new kind of coronavirus. David Guttman and John Stavrinides of Toronto University analyzed the proteins that make up the spike and nucleocapsid of the SARS virus, the matrix protein found on the inner surface of the viral envelope and a protein known as the replicase enzyme and found some to have evolved from mammalian coronaviruses, and others to have evolved from avian coronaviruses. The matrix and nucleocapsid proteins bore strong evidence of having evolved from avian viruses, while the replicase protein appeared to have mammalian origins. Significantly, the structure of the spike protein, which determines what hosts a virus can infect, was very similar to that of the spike protein in the coronavirus that infects cats, except for a small section of the gene that was very similar to that in an avian virus. The researchers suggested that this combination of genetic material from an avian and a mammalian virus in the viral spike was what had given the SARS virus the ability to infect humans. "The SARS virus is a mosaic, with at least two distinct evolutionary histories," they wrote. "We propose that a recombination event occurred within the S [spike] gene ... this event might have been the critical step in the switch to a human host and the subsequent emergence of this new pathogen."[40] The finding of a SARS-like virus in civet cats might indicate that the civet cat acted as a mixing vessel in which an avian and a mammalian coronavirus were combined.

Regardless of whether the SARS virus is an ancient virus that has lived in an animal host for centuries, or a more recent virus that has evolved as a result of the combination of an avian and a mammalian coronavirus, eradicating it will be next to impossible. If an animal that acts as the virus' natural reservoir in the wild is identified, eradicating the virus would involve slaughtering an entire animal species. If it is indeed a recombinant virus, then it might well exist in a variety of animals and birds, also making eradication impossible.

Finding the source of the SARS virus in nature and discovering its route of transmission is essential to prevent fresh outbreaks of the disease. If the SARS virus is passed from civet cats to humans in animal markets in southern China, then regulating these markets and testing the animals sold in them is a step forward in preventing a resurgence of the disease.

But this won't be easy. Immediately after the release of the finding that the coronavirus was present in civet cats, provincial authorities across China banned the sale of civet cats and over 50 other wild animal species and tightened up regulations on the animal trade. But presumably under pressure from farmers and other commercial interests, by the end of July, the ban had been lifted. The Guangdong provincial forestry department, which regulates the animal trade, decided that animals bred in captivity, like the civet cat, could go back on sale. The lifting of the ban followed a meeting of experts that found there was no evidence linking SARS to the banned animal species.[41] Technically, it is true that the studies do not prove the SARS virus passed from civet cats, or from any other animal species, to humans. But Guan Yi's study did strongly indicate that a very similar virus has been passing from civet cats and other animals to humans, and that this was possibly the source of the SARS epidemic.

In June, the China Agricultural University released the findings of a study that sampled 65 different animals from all over China, including civet cats, monkeys, bats and pigs, but found no evidence that any of them harboured the SARS coronavirus. But they did find three new kinds of coronaviruses in civet cats and hares, indicating again that the civet cat was a possible route of transmission from animals to humans.

The reappearance of isolated cases of SARS in Guangdong in January 2004 convinced the Guangdong authorities that despite the economic cost to market traders and animal breeders, the wild animal trade had to be stopped. The provincial government ordered a mass cull of civet cats, badgers and racoon dogs and a ban on their sale. Nearly 4000 animals were killed through drowning or electrocution. Theories linking civet cats to SARS were strengthened when traces of the SARS virus were discovered in a restaurant in Guangzhou where civet cats and other wild animal species were served. A waitress from the restaurant was one of those who came down with SARS in January 2004.

The culling of civet cats and restricting the trade in wild animals will act as a brake on one possible route of viral transmission from animals to humans. But experiments have shown that the SARS coronavirus is able to infect a wide range of animals, including rats and domestic cats.[42] If the coronavirus establishes itself in domestic animals, then the only protection would be an effective vaccine for both humans and domestic animals.

It is also possible that if SARS does become an increasingly common disease, its symptoms might become increasingly milder. The three people who contracted SARS in Guangdong in January 2004 had symptoms that were noticeably milder than those in SARS cases a year earlier. Their fever lasted for a shorter time, and the lungs did not deteriorate in the same way. The disease also appeared to be less infectious. None of the three cases passed it on to their family members or to anyone else with whom they had been in contact.

6

CONCLUSION

IN 1918, a virulent new influenza virus erupted in a war-torn world and swept across the globe, mowing down healthy men and women with a swiftness with which doctors were unable to cope. By the time the influenza epidemic ended a year later, it had killed between 20 and 40 million people, more than double the 10 million who died in World War I.

No one is sure when, where or how this epidemic arose.[1] It was widely known as the Spanish flu after 8 million Spaniards, including nearly a third of the population of Madrid, were laid low, but it did not originate in Spain. The epidemic swept the world in two waves: a mild form of the illness reported in the US in early 1918, followed by a more lethal wave in the second half of the same year.

One of the earliest reported outbreaks occurred at a US military post, Camp Funston in Kansas, where on a May morning in 1918, 100 soldiers fell sick with symptoms of influenza. In that month, the same illness appeared in other military camps across the US. The disease was mild, producing symptoms no more serious than the aches, pains and fever associated with an ordinary flu. Doctors thought little of it, and the men quickly recovered. But some soldiers were still sick when they were shipped off to Europe to fight in the war against Germany, and may have taken the disease with them across the Atlantic. The flu soon spread through the battlefields of Europe, striking down combatants on both sides.

But the full horror of the disease would not be felt until a second wave of infections hit the US in the latter half of that year. Soldiers returning from Europe brought back a new, more virulent form of the disease, which swept rapidly across the country. Once again, many of those who caught the virus recovered as they would from an ordinary flu. But in a number of cases, the symptoms worsened, leading to rapid death. The speed at which the disease killed its victims was astounding.

An army doctor struggling with the epidemic at Camp Devens, a US military post in Massachusetts, described how quickly his men were dying:

> Two hours after admission they have the Mahogany spots over the cheek bones, and a few hours later you can begin to see the Cyanosis extending from their ears and spreading all over the face until it is hard to distinguish the coloured men from the white. It is only a matter of a few hours then until death comes, and it is simply a struggle for air until they suffocate. It is horrible.[2]

Anecdotes were told of people leaving for work in the morning, developing the flu and dying by the end of the same day. The victims' last few hours were agonizing: their lungs would fill with blood-tinged fluid, and a bloody saliva would dribble from their lips as they suffocated to death. The disease appeared to be even more devastating than the European Black Death, and for a while it seemed as though it would succeed in doing what the artillery shells, bullets, bayonets and mustard gas of the war had failed to do: shake the foundations of modern, industrialized civilization. "If the epidemic continues its mathematical rate of acceleration, civilization could easily disappear from the earth," observed Victor Vaughan, a doctor at the forefront of the fight against the disease in the US.[3] In Philadelphia, one of the first cities to be hit by the epidemic, funeral homes were unable to cope with the number of deaths. In the city morgue, bodies were "covered only with dirty and often bloodstained sheets. Most were unembalmed and without ice. Some were mortifying and emitting a nauseating stench."[4]

The disease seemed incurable. No medicines worked, and all doctors could do was watch helplessly as patients died before their eyes. Victor Vaughan wrote, "The saddest part of my life was when I witnessed the hundreds of deaths of soldiers in the Army camps and did not know what to do. At that moment I decided never again to prate about the great achievements of medical science and to humbly admit our dense ignorance in this case."[5] Home grown remedies were developed in an attempt to fill the gaps left by medicine. Typical was the advice dispensed by the *News of the World* newspaper: "Wash inside nose with soap and water each night and morning; force yourself to sneeze night and morning, then breathe deeply; do not wear a muffler; take sharp walks regularly and walk home from work; eat plenty of porridge."[6]

By the second half of 1918, the disease had spread around the world, carried by the movement of troops to and from the battlefields of Europe. North Africa, India, the Philippines and China were all affected. India was among the worst hit, with an estimated 15–20 million deaths. In the Philippines, 40 percent of the population was infected. Then, almost as suddenly as it had arrived, in the second half of 1919, the epidemic died out, after having taken more lives than five years of warfare had. Nearly a billion people, or half the world's population at the time, were estimated to have been infected by the virus.[7]

The 1918 epidemic has largely passed out of living memory, and the devastation it wrought can only be guessed at from the written accounts left by those who experienced its horrors. We read these accounts with a certain complacency. Surely if the same thing were to happen today, we would know how to protect ourselves better than our forefathers did. After all, medicine has progressed immeasurably since the early decades of the 20th century, when antiviral drugs and vaccines against influenza had not yet been developed.

Our complacency is misplaced. Scientists believe that a devastating new form of flu could erupt at any time, and unless the world is prepared for it, the loss of life and the impact on the global economy could be catastrophic. Neither will modern medicine offer much help. Despite the advances in medical science over the last century, there is no real cure for influenza. Antiviral drugs can alleviate some of the symptoms, but do not offer protection against the disease. Vaccination is the only sure method of protecting people against influenza. But existing vaccines will not work against a new influenza virus, so a new vaccine will have to be tailor-made for the new virus. This will be an epidemic against which we will find it hard to defend ourselves.

When the first reports of the SARS outbreak in southern China reached the outside world, scientists initially took this as the beginning of the new global flu pandemic that they had been expecting. When the disease turned out not to be flu, there was general relief. However terrible SARS might be, it is not as terrible as a global influenza epidemic caused by a new flu virus would be. SARS infected slightly more than 8000 people globally and caused 1707 deaths. A new influenza pandemic could cause as many as 207 000 deaths and over 700 000 hospitalizations in the US alone. The cost of dealing with such a pandemic is estimated at between US$71 and $166 billion.[8] The World Health Organization (WHO) estimates that in the industrialized world alone, up to 650 000 people could die and as many as 2.3 million people would need to be hospitalized over a two-year period. The impact of the pandemic in developing countries would be far greater.[9] As Klaus Stohr, the coordinator of the WHO's global influenza surveillance programme, put it, "Compared with a flu pandemic, SARS will be something to smile about."[10]

It is difficult to get alarmed about an illness as common and seemingly harmless as the flu. But the disease that scientists are worried about would not be caused by any of the normal flu viruses, but by a new, mutant form of the virus. What makes influenza so terrible is its ability to reinvent itself every few decades as new lethal strains of the influenza virus emerge. The last century saw three global influenza pandemics, in 1918, 1957 and 1968, each of which was caused by a new strain of the virus. The world of the influenza virus is somewhat like a politically unstable country: there are numerous pretenders jostling for power, and every once in a while, one of them overthrows the ruler and holds power for a brief period before being overthrown in turn. Thus, in 1918, a strain of the virus known as H1N1 emerged, causing the great post-war pandemic and becoming the dominant human influenza strain. Then in the 1957 pandemic, a new strain known as H2N2 swept the world, causing several million deaths and displacing H1N1 as the main human influenza strain. In 1968, a new strain, H3N2, emerged to become the dominant strain, a position it continues to hold. It has been more than three decades since H3N2 emerged, and scientists believe that the arrival of a new influenza strain is imminent.

To understand why, it is necessary to take a brief look into the world of the influenza virus. The natural hosts of the influenza virus are thought to be aquatic birds, and over centuries, the virus has lived and evolved in the guts of these birds, causing them no harm.[11] Over time, different strains of the virus emerged and moved to other avian and mammalian hosts, including human beings.

Among other defining features, different strains of the influenza virus can be distinguished by variations in the two proteins, haemagglutinin and neuraminidase, that appear as tiny spike-like projections on the virus' surface under an electron microscope. The virus uses these projections to latch onto cells and cause infections. Fifteen haemagglutinin and nine neuraminidase subtypes have been identified so far in influenza viruses, and viruses are named according to their haemagglutinin and neuraminidase subtypes: H1N1, H2N2, H3N2 and so on.

All viruses, as indeed all living things, evolve in response to changes in their environment. But in addition to this normal evolutionary process, the influenza virus is capable of changing dramatically through a process of genetic re-assortment. Influenza viruses carry their genetic code in eight segments of RNA. This segmented structure allows different strains of the virus to swap genes among themselves, often creating versions of the virus that are totally new. This random swapping of genes does not necessarily lead to viable new forms of the virus. But every few decades, it does result in a virus that is viable and has the ability to cause severe disease in human beings. When this happens, the result is a pandemic. The new virus sweeps through human populations because people have no immunity to it.

The three new influenza viruses that afflicted the world in the last century resulted from the mixing of genes found in bird and animal flu viruses with human flu viruses to produce a lethal new strain. In the 1957 and 1968 pandemics, avian flu genes, possibly from aquatic birds, mixed with the human influenza virus to produce a new strain.[12] In the case of the 1918 epidemic, analysis of the virus recovered from the bodies of victims has failed to show conclusively how the virus originated. The 1918 virus is very similar to an influenza virus that was causing swine flu in pigs at the same time, and one possibility is that pigs were an intermediate host in which avian and human influenza viruses met and swapped genes.[13] The 1957 and 1968 influenza viruses are also believed to have originated from the mixing of human and avian flu viruses in pigs. The new virus would then have passed from pigs to humans.

The farms of southern China, where pigs, ducks, chickens and humans live cheek by jowl, and its market places, where live chicken, ducks, geese and game birds are stocked together, provide an ideal environment for different strains of influenza viruses to meet and mix. The viruses that caused two of the global influenza pandemics in the last century, the Asian flu of 1957, and the Hong Kong flu of 1968, both originated in southern China.

The 1997 bird flu outbreak in Hong Kong was seen by many as the first warning sign that a new influenza virus was on its way. That spring, an outbreak of avian influenza caused by a H5N1 virus killed some 5000 chickens in farms in Hong Kong. At first, this did not cause any great alarm, because it was widely believed that avian influenza viruses could not be transmitted directly to humans. But in May that year, a 3-year-old boy died of complications after a severe bout of flu. Tests showed that he had not been infected by a human flu virus, but rather by an H5N1 avian flu virus that was nearly identical genetically to the virus killing chickens in Hong Kong.[14] This was the first known incident in which an avian flu virus jumped directly from birds to cause disease in humans. Analysis of the virus provided a glimpse into the complex genetic exchanges going on in the avian influenza world. The H5N1 virus was a new strain that had arisen due to genetic re-assortment between goose and quail viruses. The haemagglutinin, or H gene, had come from a goose virus; the internal genes had come from an H9N2 quail virus; and the neuraminidase, or N gene, had come from an H6N1 quail virus. The H5N1 virus was the result of three other viruses recombining to create a new virus that was lethal to both chickens and humans.[15]

Eighteen people contracted H5N1 influenza in Hong Kong in 1997, and their illness provided a glimpse of what a new influenza pandemic could be like. Their symptoms were more severe than those of normal influenza, and the death rate was high: 6 of the 18 cases, or a third, died. Fortunately, the virus had not quite yet adapted to its human host enough to transmit easily between humans. Each of the 18 victims had caught the virus directly from infected poultry. The real worry though, was that as more and more humans caught H5N1 influenza, the virus would adapt to humans and become more transmissible. Once that happened, a new influenza pandemic was inevitable.

The normal human influenza virus, H3N2, was also circulating in Hong Kong at the time. If people became infected with both viruses, the avian virus would quickly acquire the genes from the human influenza virus that would allow it to transmit between human beings. To prevent the avian virus from spreading any further in the human population and mixing with the human influenza virus, the Hong Kong government culled 1.5 million chickens as well as a smaller number of ducks and geese being bred on farms throughout the territory, removing the source of the H5N1 virus in Hong Kong. This move probably averted an incipient pandemic.

But it was only a temporary reprieve. The 1997 incident was like the first rumblings of a volcano about to erupt. More rumblings were to follow. Two years later, an avian flu virus was again transmitted to humans in Hong Kong when two children fell ill with an H9N2 virus that appeared to have originated in quails. Then, in late February 2003, the H5N1 virus reappeared briefly, killing a 33-year-old Hong Kong man and his 9-year-old son, both of whom probably caught the virus during a visit to China.

Southern China and Hong Kong are traditionally regarded as the region where a new influenza virus is likely to emerge. But in March 2003, it became apparent that a new flu virus could appear anywhere in the world. Chicken farms in the Netherlands and later in Belgium were hit by a strain of the H7N7 virus that also infected humans.[16] At least 80 people became infected with the virus, which fortunately only caused conjunctivitis and mild illness in most cases. The only death was of a 57-year-old veterinarian, who had caught the disease while visiting a poultry farm. Though the symptoms were mild, the dangers were obvious: if the virus was given more opportunity to transmit to humans, it was only a matter of time before it infected someone who was also carrying the normal human flu virus. As Albert Osterhaus of the Erasmus University in Rotterdam commented at the time: "It's an explosive mix. If avian flu is present in people at the same time as the human influenza virus, we could have the start of a pandemic."[17] The only way to stop the avian virus from spreading any further among humans was by eliminating it from the poultry population. The Dutch government did what the Hong Kong government had done earlier, and slaughtered several million chickens to end the epidemic.

Then later that year, the H5N1 avian flu virus reappeared, but this time in Asia. The new outbreak was first reported in early December 2003 in South Korea, when nearly 20 000 chickens died on a farm in Emsung district near Seoul. The virus also emerged in Thailand, Vietnam and Indonesia at around the same time, but went unreported.

There were no human cases of influenza in South Korea, where infected farms were quarantined and nearly 2 million chicken and ducks were slaughtered to prevent the disease from spreading. Among the casualties was the country's largest duck processor, Fine Korea, which declared bankruptcy after the cull and the decline in duck meat sales.[18] The disease then surfaced in Japan, in the first such outbreak the country had experienced since 1925. The culling of over 30 000 chickens was successful in containing the outbreak. In Japan too, there were no human cases.

But in early January 2004, the inevitable happened and the virus began to infect human beings. The disease broke out in Vietnam, and children who lived on or near farms with infected chickens came down with a severe influenza caused by the H5N1 virus. The same pattern appeared in Thailand. The virus, though lethal, was unable to transmit easily between humans, so the number of cases was relatively small.

Initial analysis of the virus showed that its genetic structure had evolved since the 1997 and 2003 outbreaks. It had still not adapted to transmitting between humans, but it caused a higher mortality rate than the 1997 virus. Of the 31 human cases that had been reported in Thailand and Vietnam by the end of February 2004, 22 had died — a mortality rate of over 70 percent. This was more than double the mortality rate in the 1997 outbreak in Hong Kong, and indicated how lethal a global pandemic caused by this virus would be.

This was the third time that the H5N1 virus had infected human beings since 1997. Each outbreak was another opportunity for the H5N1 virus to acquire the genetic information it needed to transmit easily between humans and cause a global pandemic. There will be other outbreaks, and influenza watchers believe it is only a matter of time before the virus, or perhaps some other strain of avian or animal influenza virus, acquires the capacity to transmit readily between humans and cause a global pandemic. And most scientists are convinced that when this does happen, the world will be woefully unprepared to fight it.[19]

SARS was a dress rehearsal for the more serious threat posed by a new influenza pandemic. The stresses that public health systems as well as individual doctors and nurses experienced during the SARS epidemic are a warning that even in some of the most advanced countries in the world, hospitals will find it difficult to cope with an influenza pandemic. As Gro Harlem Brundtland, the former Director-General of the WHO, pointed out:

SARS has exposed serious weaknesses in health systems around the world. The disease places an enormous burden on health services in terms of infection control, isolation, long periods of intensive care and the demands of contact tracing and follow up or quarantine. Even in areas with highly developed social services, the burden of coping with SARS, the number of hospital patients and health workers who became infected, often brought health systems to the verge of collapse.[20]

The numbers of SARS cases in 2003 was a modest 8000 across the world. In the case of an influenza pandemic, the numbers would be in the millions.[21] The pressures that medical staff would be under can only be imagined. Even a disease as contagious as SARS saw doctors and nurses fall ill themselves, increasing the strain on public health systems. Influenza is far more easily transmissible than SARS, possibly placing medical staff at even greater risk.[22] Similarly, intensive care units in SARS-affected cities were stretched to the limits by numbers of patients that would be small compared to those during an influenza epidemic.

The only way to prevent an influenza pandemic is through large scale vaccination. Vaccines will have to be tailor-made for any new flu virus, and time as well as money will be a constraint. Developing the vaccine, subjecting it to clinical trials and then getting it ready for commercial production will take at least six months to a year. In this period of time, the virus would have already infected hundreds of thousands of people across the world.

Developing a vaccine for the H5N1 virus also poses technical challenges for researchers. The viruses used to develop flu vaccines are normally cultured in chicken embryos. But this technique will not work in the case of the H5N1 virus, which is lethal to chickens and kills the chick embryos in which it is supposed to grow. Researchers have to use a process known as reverse genetics to genetically tailor a virus for vaccine development that will not kill chicken embryos. Getting safety approval for a virus developed this way, as well as persuading commercial manufacturers to assume the risk of producing the vaccine, will take additional time. Even though vaccine manufacturers can use modern genetic engineering techniques to develop a vaccine, commercial production will still be based on the old-fashioned technique of growing the vaccine-producing virus in chickens' eggs. And a major constraint on vaccine production will be a shortage of eggs. Tens of millions of eggs will be required, and it will take months for companies producing the vaccine to line up the supplies of eggs needed.

Antiviral drugs, which cannot prevent the disease but might help reduce the severity of flu symptoms, will also be in short supply. Countries like the US have plans to stockpile supplies of antiviral drugs, but other countries that have not built up supplies will find the drugs hard to come by.

A global influenza pandemic will also throw into sharp relief the divisions between the wealthy and poor nations of the world in the same way that the AIDS epidemic has done. While the majority of cases will be in the poorer developing countries, the limited supplies of vaccines and antiviral drugs will go to patients in the developed world. The vaccine- and antiviral drug-producing companies are all based in the developed world, and their product is likely to be bought up by governments in these countries. As Klaus Stohr of the WHO said, "Our concern is that during an influenza pandemic influenza vaccines will not reach developing countries until developed countries would have set aside their demands because [vaccine producing] companies are there."[23]

Neither are developing countries in a position to do the detailed contingency planning that richer countries have been able to do. These plans involve decisions on the allocation of hospital beds, putting together priority lists for vaccination, stockpiling drugs, developing treatment guidelines and so on. Canada's contingency plan for a global flu pandemic, for example, includes keeping in reserve 165 portable hospitals with 33 000 beds that can be deployed anywhere in the country where extra beds are required.

Developing countries struggling with the burden of other equally pressing diseases cannot afford such contingency arrangements. As Ann-Emmanuelle Birn, a public health expert at the University of Toronto, pointed out, "It would be very difficult to ask a country like Nicaragua, where access to basic clean water is an issue, or South Africa, which is struggling with providing anti retroviral drugs to deal with AIDS ... to stop all these dire needs to cope with a potential influenza pandemic."[24]

* * *

After the SARS epidemic of 2003 ended, the question everyone asked was whether it would come back. In fact, it never really went away. The SARS virus may have stopped spreading in the human population by mid-June of that year, but it continued to exist and multiply in the animal population in southern China. Since host animals like the civet cat come into close contact with humans on breeding farms and in marketplaces, it was only a matter of time before the virus once again crossed over into the human population. Sure enough, isolated cases of SARS reappeared in China in December of that year and in January 2004. But the disease did not spread beyond a handful of cases, and there were no deaths. SARS was no longer a new disease, and doctors everywhere were alert for the first signs of its reappearance. Those who caught the disease were quickly isolated in hospital before they could pass it on.

It is unlikely that fresh outbreaks of SARS will lead to the economic and social collapse experienced in the 2003 epidemic. SARS was terrifying the first time around because it was unknown. This is no longer the case. But it is very likely that other new diseases will emerge in the decades ahead with the potential to cause at least as much human suffering as SARS did. Some of them, like AIDS, could result in long, smouldering epidemics. Others, like SARS, will die down relatively quickly, and cause little long-term damage. Whatever their nature, we can be sure that new diseases will continue to emerge. As Joshua Lederberg and others have pointed out, microbes are the only natural predators that continue to pose a threat to our survival.

We are so used to the idea that we have conquered disease that it is difficult for us to take the danger posed by the microbial world seriously. Even when we are forewarned that a lethal new disease is likely to emerge, we often find it hard to muster the collective will to take the steps necessary to protect ourselves against this threat. The H5N1 avian flu outbreak in Asia is a case in point. While rapid culling of chickens was the only way to stop the disease from spreading, governments were in general reluctant to acknowledge the existence of a serious health threat and to order the slaughter of birds. And there were good reasons for this reluctance. The livelihood of hundreds of thousands of farmers was at risk, and many of the poorer countries did not have the means to compensate farmers adequately for their loss. In addition, there were the follow-on effects of losing export markets and being shunned by tourists and business visitors. It all came down to a question of choosing between two risks: the risk of loss of livelihood and economic distress against the risk of a major new epidemic. For most people, and for governments as well, the loss of livelihood seems a more immediate threat than the possibility of being ravaged by a lethal new disease.

If SARS has helped to awaken people and governments across the world, particularly in Asia, of the devastation that a new disease can cause, then at least some small good would have come out of the epidemic. But it is not apparent that this has happened. Governments and people are sensitive to the dangers of SARS, and willing to do whatever it takes to prevent a new SARS epidemic. But like generals who base their battle plans on the last war that they fought, focusing narrowly on SARS will almost guarantee that we are caught unprepared when real danger erupts.

The real danger is not the return of SARS. It is the eruption of the next disease caused by a new virus. The emergence of an influenza pandemic caused by a new flu virus is almost certain. But when it does come, most of the world will once again be caught unawares. Even among the wealthy nations, only Canada has an influenza pandemic preparedness plan that ensures vaccination for the entire population. No country has prepared stockpiles of antiviral drugs that could be used to reduce the severity of the illness. At a global level, no plans have been made to ensure that poorer countries will have access to vaccines and antiviral drugs.

SARS offered us valuable lessons on how to fight new global diseases. It demonstrated the importance of early, transparent disease reporting, without which a new disease can spread rapidly across the world. It showed us that global cooperation on many levels is required to control a disease. Scientists and doctors need to share information and collaborate to find the best ways of treating a new disease and preventing its spread. Governments have to recognize that a disease in any one part of the world is a threat to every other part of the world, and work together to fight common threats. The test of how well these lessons have been learned will be when the next new disease emerges in the not too distant future.

Appendix 1

THE SARS EPIDEMIC OF 2002–2003
A Chronology

2002

November 16. A 46-year-old village committee official is admitted to hospital in Foshan, Guangdong province, with a mysterious respiratory ailment which his wife and other family members also develop. He has no history of travel outside Foshan in the weeks before he fell ill, nor has he been in contact with wild animals that could have passed on the coronavirus. He recovers and is discharged on January 8, 2003. Now recognized as the first known case of SARS.

December 10. A 34-year-old restaurant chef, Huang Xingchu, is admitted to hospital in Heyuan with a respiratory illness that does not respond to normal treatment. He cooks wild animal meat but is not involved in killing animals. His condition deteriorates, and he is transferred to the Guangzhou Military General Hospital on December 17, recovers, and is discharged on January 10, 2003. Seven medical workers in Heyuan fall ill later in the month

December 21. A 26-year-old male factory worker falls ill in Jiangmen, Guangdong province, with a respiratory illness that does not respond to normal treatment.

December 26. A 30-year-old male who works as a chef in Zhongshan, Guangdong province, is admitted to hospital. He infects 12 others including two relatives and 10 health care workers.

2003

January 2. Public panic in Heyuan as people hear about medical staff falling ill. Heyuan authorities inform the provincial centre for disease control in Guangzhou and appeal for public calm. The provincial centre for disease control sends investigators to Heyuan. A 49-year-old government official is admitted to the Guangdong Traditional Chinese Medicine Hospital in Guangzhou where he infects seven health care workers.

January 18. Health authorities in Zhongshan inform provincial centre for disease control that 28 people including 13 health care workers have come down with a respiratory illness. News of the illness causes public alarm in Zhongshan, and people queue for medicines and vinegar.

January 21. A team from the provincial centre for diseases control and the national centre for disease control in Beijing arrive in Zhongshan to investigate the epidemic.

January 22. A 49-year-old Hong Kong woman falls ill after visiting her mother in the mainland. She is admitted to hospital in Hong Kong and dies on February 3. Retrospective analysis of her serum samples shows she had been infected with SARS, making her one of the first cases in Hong Kong. A nurse who looked after her was also infected.

January 23. The investigating team in Zhongshan produce a five-page report describing the disease as "atypical pneumonia." The report and a letter warning major hospitals in the region about the disease is released on this day. However, some hospitals appear to have received the notification only a week or so later.

January 28. Hospital workers begin to fall ill in Guangzhou. Seven hospital workers at the Guangdong Provincial Hospital for Traditional Chinese medicine fall ill.

January 30. Zhou Zuofeng, the first SARS "super spreader," is admitted to the Second Affiliated Hospital, Zhongshan Medical University, Guangzhou.

January 31. As the number of cases in Guangzhou increase, health authorities decide to centralize treatment by channelling all suspected SARS cases to seven hospitals in the city.

February 10. Hong Kong media report a mysterious disease in Guangdong province causing panic. The Department of Health in Hong Kong tries to contact the authorities in Guangdong, but receives no reply.

February 10. The WHO Regional Office in Manila asks the Chinese Ministry of Health for more information about reports of the illness in Guangdong.

February 11. Guangdong provincial health authorities hold a press conference acknowledging the disease and stating that there had been 305 cases and five deaths until February 9. The health authorities said the epidemic was under control, and there was no need for panic. The same day the WHO receives reports from the Chinese Ministry of Health.

February 12. Two researchers from the University of Hong Kong travel unofficially to Guangzhou to get samples from mainland patients. Their main concern is to see whether this disease has been caused by a virulent new influenza virus. The WHO global influenza network is also waiting to see what they come back with.

February 20. After human deaths from bird flu are reported in Hong Kong, the WHO becomes more anxious to investigate the outbreak in Guangdong. The WHO Regional Director in Manila, Shigeru Omi, writes to the Chinese authorities asking for permission to send an investigative team. In Washington, the US Health Secretary, Tommy Thompson, also urges the visiting Chinese Deputy Minister of Health to allow the WHO request. China gives permission.

February 21. Liu Jianlun, a 64-year-old professor of nephrology from Guangzhou, arrives in Hong Kong for his nephew's wedding. He and his wife check into the Metropole Hotel, but the next day he feels unwell and admits himself to Kwong Wah Hospital. At the Metropole Hotel, he infects a group of travellers from different countries, and triggers a global epidemic.

February 23-25. Guests from the Metropole Hotel who had been infected by Liu carry the SARS virus to different parts of the world. A 78-year-old Canadian woman, Kwan Sui Chu, takes it to Toronto: Johnny Chen, a Chinese American businessman, takes it to Hanoi; and three young women take the disease to Singapore.

February 23. A two-member WHO team arrives in Beijing but is not given permission to visit Guangdong. They leave China after two weeks in Beijing waiting for permission.

February 28. Carlo Urbani, a specialist at the WHO office in Hanoi, is asked by the French Hospital in Hanoi for advice on how to treat Johnny Chen. Urbani is alarmed by the severity of the symptoms, and the way it spreads among doctors and health care workers. His reports put the WHO on alert.

March 1. Esther Mok, a 26-year-old guest at the Metropole Hotel, becomes Singapore's index patient for SARS and is admitted to Tan Tock Seng Hospital.

March 4. A 26-year-old Hong Kong man, who had visited a friend at the Metropole Hotel in February, is admitted to Ward 8 A at the Prince of Wales Hospital with a severe respiratory ailment. He triggers an epidemic in the hospital, which spreads to the community.

March 5. Beijing receives its first SARS case, when a businesswoman from Shanxi province who fell ill after a trip to Guangdong is hospitalized at a People's Liberation Army hospital. The Chinese National People's Congress also begins a crucial session to appoint a new government.

March 10. Doctors and nurses at the Prince of Wales Hospital fall ill in unusually large numbers. The hospital authorities inform the Hong Kong Department of Health.

March 12. Hong Kong health authorities inform WHO about the outbreak at the Prince of Wales Hospital. Alarmed by the cases from Hanoi and Hong Kong, the WHO puts out an alert warning the world about the outbreaks of atypical pneumonia, recommending that patients with suspicious symptoms be isolated.

March 15. The WHO steps up its warnings and issues an emergency travel advisory, after the Singapore health authorities inform the WHO that a doctor with SARS symptoms was travelling on a flight from New York to Singapore and needed to be hospitalized. The WHO names the disease Severe Acute Respiratory Syndrome (SARS).
Canada reports 8 cases and two deaths from the disease.
Singapore reports 16 cases.

March 16. Over 150 suspect and probable cases reported to the WHO from all around the world.

March 17. China provides a brief report to the WHO stating that the outbreak in Guangdong had tapered off. The WHO sets up a collaborative network of laboratories around the world to detect the agent causing SARS and develop reliable diagnostic tests. A team from the University of Hong Kong isolates what it believes to be the causal agent for SARS, and begins tests to confirm this.

March 18–19. Chinese University of Hong Kong and laboratories in Germany, Canada and Singapore announce the virus causing SARS might be a paramyxovirus. At the University of Hong Kong, this is ruled out, and tests continue on the virus they have isolated.

March 21. Malik Peiris of the University of Hong Kong emails the WHO laboratory network to inform them that his team has isolated the SARS virus. The University of Hong Kong team also devises a basic diagnostic test based on the isolated virus.

March 23. A WHO team arrives in Beijing and asks to travel to Guangdong province.

March 26. The first official acknowledgement of SARS in Beijing comes in a dispatch from Xinhua news agency which says the Chinese capital has a few "imported" cases.

March 27. Various labs in the WHO network confirm the University of Hong Kong's findings and identify the SARS virus as a previously unknown coronavirus.

March 29. Carlo Urbani, the WHO doctor who alerted the world to SARS, dies in Bangkok.

March 31. Isolation order imposed on Amoy Gardens to prevent the further spread of SARS in the housing complex.

April 2. The WHO issues an advisory recommending only essential travel to Hong Kong and Guangdong province. This is described as the most stringent travel advisory the WHO has ever issued, and follows evidence that travellers from Singapore, Beijing, and Taiwan had caught SARS in Hong Kong and taken it back with them.

April 3. A WHO team arrives in Guangdong. In Beijing, Health Minister Zhang Wenkang tells a televised press conference that the city had 12 cases of SARS, but the disease was under control.

April 6. A Finnish staff member of the International Labour Organization dies of SARS in Beijing, after catching the disease from a fellow passenger on a flight from Bangkok.

April 16. Chinese Premier Wen Jiabao acknowledges that the situation caused by SARS in China is "extremely grave." The next day President Hu Jintao calls a Politbureau meeting to emphasize the gravity of the situation.

April 20. Minister of Health Zhang Wenkang and the Mayor of Beijing are removed from their posts, apparently for having covered up the extent of the SARS outbreak. Authorities disclose 339 previously unreported cases of SARS. China becomes more open about the disease.

April 23. The WHO issues travel advisories for Toronto, Beijing and Shanxi province in China.

April 28. After reporting no fresh outbreaks of SARS for two weeks, Vietnam becomes the first country to contain the disease.

May 3. The WHO sends a team to Taiwan, as the number of cases begins to grow.

May 22. A fresh outbreak of SARS occurs in a Toronto hospital, a week after it was certified free of the disease by the WHO.

May 23. Researchers in the University of Hong Kong announce they have found a virus very similar to the SARS virus among civet cats and a few other species of animals in China that are sold for human consumption.

May 31. Singapore is declared free of SARS.

June 23. Hong Kong is free of SARS.

June 24. Beijing is declared free of SARS, and the WHO removes its recommendation against travel to the city.

July 2. Toronto is declared free of SARS after its second outbreak.

July 5. Taiwan is declared SARS free, and the WHO declares the epidemic has been contained worldwide.

Appendix 2

SARS CASES WORLDWIDE
November 1, 2002 – July 31, 2003

(Source: World Health Organization)

Areas	Female	Male	Total	Median age	Number of deaths[a]	Case fatality ratio	Number of imported cases (%)	Number of HCW affected (%)	Date onset first probable case	Date onset onset last probable cases
Australia	4	2	6	15 (1–45)	0	0	6 (100)	1 (16)	26-Feb-03	1-Apr-03
Canada	151	100	251	49 (1–98)	43	17	5 (2)	109 (43)	23-Feb-03	12-Jun-03
China	2674	2607	5327[b]	Pending	349	7	Not Applicable	1002 (19)	16-Nov-02	3-Jun-03
China, Hong Kong SAR	977	778	1755	40 (0–100)	299	17	Not	386 (22)	15-Feb-03	31-May-03
China, Macao SAR	0	1	1	28	0	0	1 (100)	0 (0)	5-May-03	5-May-03
China, Taiwan	218	128	346[c]	42 (0–93)	37	11	21 (6)	68 (20)	25-Feb-03	15-Jun-03
France	1	6	7	49 (26–56)	1	14	7 (100)	2 (29)[d]	21-Mar-03	3-May-03
Germany	4	5	9	44 (4–73)	0	0	9 (100)	1 (11)	9-Mar-03	6-May-03
India	0	3	3	25 (25–30)	0	0	3 (100)	0 (0)	25-Apr-03	6-May-03
Indonesia	0	2	2	56 (47–65)	0	0	2 (100)	0 (0)	6-Apr-03	17-Apr-03
Italy	1	3	4	30.5 (25–54)	0	0	4 (100)	0 (0)	12-Mar-03	20-Apr-03
Kuwait	1	0	1	50	0	0	1 (100)	0 (0)	9-Apr-03	9-Apr-03
Malaysia	1	4	5	30 (26–84)	2	40	5 (100)	0 (0)	14-Mar-03	22-Apr-03
Mongolia	8	1	9	32 (17–63)	0	0	8 (89)	0 (0)	31-Mar-03	6-May-03
New Zealand	1	0	1	67	0	0	1 (100)	0 (0)	20-Apr-03	20-Apr-03
Philippines	8	6	14	41 (29–73)	2	14	7 (50)	4 (29)	25-Feb-03	5-May-03
Republic of Ireland	0	1	1	56	0	0	1 (100)	0 (0)	27-Feb-03	27-Feb-03
Republic of Korea	0	3	3	40 (20–80)	0	0	3 (100)	0 (0)	25-Apr-03	10-May-03
Romania	0	1	1	52	0	0	1 (100)	0 (0)	19-Mar-03	19-Mar-03

(Table to be continued)

(Table continued)

Areas	Female	Male	Total	Median age	Number of deaths	Case fatality ratio	Number of imported cases (%)	Number of HCW affected (%)	Date onset first probable case	Date onset last probable cases
Russian Federation	0	1	1	25	0	0	Not Applicable	0 (0)	5-May-03	5-May-03
Singapore	161	77	238	3 (1–90)	33	14	8 (3)	97 (41)	25-Feb-03	5-May-03
South Africa	0	1	1	62	1	100	1 (100)	0 (0)	3-Apr-03	3-Apr-03
Spain	0	1	1	33	0	0	1 (100)	0 (0)	26-Mar-03	26-Mar-03
Sweden	3	2	5	43 (33–55)	0	0	5 (100)	0 (0)	28-Mar-03	23-Apr-03
Switzerland	0	1	1	35	0	0	1 (100)	0 (0)	9-Mar-03	9-Mar-03
Thailand	5	4	9	42(2–79)	2	22	9 (100)	1 (11)c	11-Mar-03	27-May-03
United Kingdom	2	2	4	59(28–74)	0	0	4 (100)	0 (0)	1-Mar-03	1-Apr-03
United States	14	15	29	33 (0–83)	0	0	28 (97)d	0 (0)	24-Feb-03	13-Jul-03e
Viet Nam	39	24	63	43 (20–76)	5	8	1 (2)	36 (57)	23-Feb-03	14-Apr-03
Total			**8098**		**774**	**9.6**		**143**	**1707 (21)**	

[a.] Includes only cases whose death is attributed to SARS.

[b.] Case classification by sex is unknown for 46 cases.

[c.] Since July 11, 2003, 325 cases have been discarded in Taiwan. Laboratory information was insufficient or incomplete for 135 discarded cases, of which 101 died.

[d.] Includes HCWs who acquired illness in other areas.

[e.] Due to differences in case definitions, the United States has reported probable cases of SARS with onsets of illness after July 5, 2003.

NOTES

CHAPTER 1

1. William Ho, "Messages from the War Front," *Hong Kong Medical Diary* 2003, 8: 13–14.

2. Chua Jui Meng, Opening Speech, WHO Global Meeting on SARS, Kuala Lumpur, June 17, 2003, http://www.who.int/csr/sars/conference/june_2003/materials/presentations/meng/en.

3. Gro Harlem Brundtland, WHO Global Meeting on SARS, Kuala Lumpur, June 17, 2003. http://www.who.int/csr/sars/conference/june_2003/materials/presentations/brundtland/en.

4. Joshua Lederberg, "Mankind Had a Near Miss From a Mystery Pandemic," *The Washington Post*, Sept 7, 1968.

5. For a description of the disease and its symptoms see http://www.cdc.gov/ncidod/dvrd/spb/mnpages/dispages/marburg.htm.

6. Joshua Lederberg, "Viruses and Humankind: Intracellular Symbiosis and Evolutionary Competition," *Emerging Viruses*, ed. Stephen S Morse, New York: Oxford University Press, 1993.

7. See note 4.

8. Cited in Laurie Garret, *The Coming Plague.Newly Emerging Diseases in a World out of Balance.* New York: Penguin, 1995. p. 33

9. For a survey of the re-emergence of infectious diseases see Mary Kay Kindhauser, ed., *Global defence against the infectious disease,* Geneva: WHO, 2003.

10. For a well-written account of the rise of resistance to antibiotics see *Overcoming Antimicrobial Resistance*, Geneva: WHO, 2000.

11. Among these were Richard M Krause, *The Restless Tide: The Persistent Challenge of the Microbial World*, Washington DC: National Foundation for Infectious Diseases, 1981, and Joshua Lederberg, Robert E Shope and Stanley C Oaks Jr, eds., *Emerging Infectious Diseases: Microbial Threats to Health in the United States*, Washington DC: National Academy Press, 1992.

12. Dorothy H Crawford, *The Invisible Enemy: A Natural History of Viruses*, Oxford: Oxford University Press, 2000.

13. See note 6.

14. For an analysis of human changes to the environment and other factors that lead to the emergence of new viral diseases see Stephen S Morse, "Examining the Origins of Emerging Viruses," *Emerging Viruses*, ed. Stephen S Morse, New York: Oxford University Press, 1993.

15. For a concise summary of the origins of AIDS see Crawford op cit.

16. For a description of the Nipah outbreak see the report by the United Nations Food and Agriculture Organization at http://www.fao.org/DOCREP/005/AC449E/ac449e04.htm.

17. Peter Fritsch, "Containing the Outbreak. Scientists Search for Human Hand Behind Outbreak of Jungle Virus," *Wall Street Journal*, Eastern Edition, June 19, 2003.

18. Mary Kay Kindhauser, op cit., p. 75.

19. http://www.rzu2u.com/gambian.html.

20. Texas Department of Health, News Release, June 11, 2003, http://www.tdh.state.tx.us/news/b_new481.htm.

21. Graeme Zilenski, "Monkeypox virus causes big stir on farm," *Milwaukee Journal Sentinel*, June 10, 2003.

22. "Pet Prairie Dogs Suspected in U.S Monkeypox Outbreak," *Scientific American*, June 10, 2003.

23. Rob Stein, "West Nile Spreading Rapidly," *The Washington Post*, July 16, 2003.

24. A superb account of the role of disease in influencing human history can be had in William H McNeill, *Plagues and Peoples*, New York: Anchor Press/Doubleday, 1976.

CHAPTER **2**

1. Zeng Wenqiong, *Heroes of anti-SARS battle*, Guangzhou: Guangzhou Publishing Company, 2003.

2. WHO Summary of probable SARS cases with onset of illness from 1 November 2002 to 31 July 2003, http://www.who.int/csr/sars/country/table2003_09_23/en.

3. Z Zhao, F Zhang, M Xu et al, "Description and clinical treatment of an early outbreak of serve acute respiratory syndrome (SARS) in Guangzhou, PR China," *Journal of Medical Microbiology* 2003, 52: 71–720.

4. Information from a confidential source.

5. The government refutes the rumour about atypical pneumonia to eliminate panic of the public", *Nanfang Daily*, February 12, 2003

6. Quoted in Gao Erqiang, "Opening up on SARS," *Shanghai Star*, May 22, 2003.

7. "SARS, a valuable lesson for the Chinese government to learn," *People's Daily*, June 9, 2003, http://english.peopledaily.com.cn/200306/08/eng20030608_117858.shtml.

8. Personal communication from Dr Fu Hualing of the Faculty of Law, the University of Hong Kong.

9. See Mary Kay Kindhauser, ed., *Global defence against the infectious disease*, Geneva: WHO, 2003, p. 65.

10. Leu Sew Ying, "Province hushed up disease to protect economy, says lawmaker," *South China Morning Post*, March 30, 2003, p. 2.

11. This account is in Zhang Shumei, *Report from the SARS frontline*, Guangzhou: Huacheng Publishing Company, 2003.

12. CCTV Interview, June 9, 2003

13. Cited in Lai Hailong, "Who Knocked Over the SARS Domino?" *Zhongguo Xinwen She* news service, June 2, 2003.

14. Ibid.

15. John Pomfret, "Signs of Improvement at Epicentre of SARS Outbreak; Province's Handling of Virus is Called Model for China," *The Washington Post*, May 4, 2003.

16. NS Zhong, BJ Zheng, YM Li et al, "Epidemiology and cause of severe acute respiratory syndrome (SARS) in Guangdong People's Republic of China in February 2003," *Lancet* 2003, 362: 13553–58.

17. CCTV Interview, June 2003

18. Interview in *Yangcheng Evening News*, June 10, 2003. English translation http://www.china.org.cn/english/2003/Jun/67051.htm

19. Wen Jiao, "Uncompromising Doctor- Zhong Nanshan", *China Daily*, May 2, 2003.

20. The struggle to save Zhou is described in Zeng Wenqiong, "Heroes of the anti-SARS battle."

21. Interview with CCTV, June 2003.

22. Zhang Jihui, "Diary of a Charge Nurse", *Nanfang Daily*, April 17, 2003

23. Interview with CCTV, June 2003

24. Matt Pottinger, "Survivors of SARS Suffer Severe Effects of Treatment," *Asian Wall Street Journal*, December 23, 2003.

25. For an analysis of the interplay between the transition of political power in China and the handling of SARS, see Joseph Fewsmith, "China's Response to SARS," *China Leadership Monitor* No 7, California: Hoover Institute.

26. Quoted in the commentary "Ailing Health System Exposed," http://www.chinaelections.org/Eng/readnews.asp?newsid={C5BF731D-93EB-4F82-8F6F-F31021859622}.

27. An edited transcript of Zhang's press conference can be found on http://www.china.org.cn.

28. John Pomfret, "Outbreak Gave China's Hu an Opening; President Responded to Pressure Inside and Outside Country on SARS," *The Washington Post*, May 13, 2003

29. John Pomfret, "China's Crisis Has a Political Edge," *The Washington Post*, April 27, 2003.

30. "A Chinese Doctor's Extraordinary April," *Sanlian Weekly* No 23, English translation, http://www.china.org.cn.

31. The English text of Jiang's letter can be found at www.china.org.cn.
32. Reported by Reuters news agency on April 16, 2003.
33. John Pomfret, "As 10 More Die, Chinese Official Terms SARS Grave Crisis; Premier Says Disease Outbreak Could Affect Nation's Stability," *The Washington Post*, April 15, 2003.

CHAPTER 3

1. Personal interview.
2. Personal interview.
3. *Report of the Hospital Authority Review Panel on the SARS Outbreak,* Hong Kong: Hospital Authority, Oct 16, 2003, http://www.ha.org.hk/sars/ps/report/reviewpanel_e.pdf.
4. See SARS Expert Committee, *SARS in Hong Kong: From Experience to Action*, Oct 2, 2003, http://www.sars-expertcom.gov.hk/english/reports/reports.html.
5. Ibid.
6. Legislative Council of Hong Kong, Minutes of the Panel on Health Service, March 28, 2003.
7. See the comments made in *Report of the Hospital Authority Review Panel on the SARS Outbreak.*
8. Reported in *SARS in Hong Kong: From Experience to Action.*
9. WHO, Press conference, Hong Kong, May 16, 2003.
10. Personal interview.
11. The clinical experience at the Prince of Wales Hospital is described in Brian Tomlinson and Clive Cockram, "SARS: experience at the Prince of Wales Hospital, Hong Kong," *Lancet* 2003, 361: 1486–1487, and Nelson Lee, David Hui, Alan Wu et al, "A Major Outbreak of Severe Acute Respiratory Syndrome in Hong Kong," *New England Journal of Medicine* 2003, 348: 1986–94.
12. Personal interview.
13. Personal interview.
14. Personal interview
15. Personal Interview
16. Ibid.
17. Personal interview.
18. Lam Shiu-kam, "Winning and Losing: the fight against SARS," *South China Morning Post*, April 9, 2003.
19. Mary Ann Benitez, "We're not to blame for SARS spread say Medics," *South China Morning Post*, April 15, 2003.
20. Personal interview.
21. Ibid.
22. Personal interview.
23. Ibid.

24. World Health Organization, Regional Office for the Western Pacific. Press Release

25. Stephen Ng, "The Mystery of Amoy Gardens," *At the Epicentre: Hong Kong and the SARS Epidemic*, ed. Christine Loh and Civic Exchange, Hong Kong: Hong Kong University Press, 2004.

26. Peter A Cameron, "The Plague Within, an Australian Doctor's Experience of SARS in Hong Kong," *Medical Journal of Australia* 2003, 178: 512–513.

27. Personal interview.

28. Mary Ann Benitez, "Hospitals restricting access to N95 masks," *South China Morning Post*, May 17 2003.

29. For the impact that public health interventions and changes in personal behaviour had on the transmission of SARS, see Steven Riley, Christophe Fraser, Christl Donnelly et al, "Transmission dynamics of the aetiological agent of Severe Acute Respiratory Syndrome (SARS) in Hong Kong. The impact of public health interventions," *Science* 2003, 300 (5627): 1961–66.

CHAPTER 4

1. This reconstruction of events at WHO headquarters is based on interviews with the WHO officials involved.

2. Ellen Nakashima, "Vietnam Took Lead in Containing SARS; Decisiveness, Luck Credited," *The Washington Post*, May 5, 2003.

3. "WHO issues a global alert about cases of atypical pneumonia." WHO press release, March 12, 2003, http://www.who.int/mediacentre/releases/2003/pr22/en.

4. Elena Cherney and Mark Heinzel, "Toronto Doctors Race to Get Handle on SARS: New Virus Caught City Off Guard in Days Before Global Health Alert," *Wall Street Journal*, April 8, 2003.

5. "Severe Acute Respiratory Syndrome — Singapore 2003," *Morbidity and Mortality Weekly Review*, Centre for Diseases Control and Prevention Atlanta, 2003, 52(18): 405–411.

6. Personal Interview

7. Personal Interview

8. Brundtland's reflections on SARS and the decisions taken by the WHO are contained in an interview she gave in June 2003 for a WHO oral history of SARS.

9. Personal interview

10. The text can be found at http://www.who.int/csr/sars/archive/2003_03_15/en.

11. Ellen Nakashima, "Vietnamese Cautiously Hail Progress on SARS; Strict Measures Planned to Prevent New Cases," *The Washington Post*, May 1, 2003.

12. Rob Stein, "Epidemic Kills Scientist Who Helped Discover It," *The Washington Post*, March 30, 2003.

13. See Lorenzo Savioli, Obituary for Carlo Urbani, *The Guardian*, April 21, 2003.
14. Ibid.
15. Personal interview.
16. Joseph Kahn, "Even in remote China, SARS arrives in force," *New York Times*, April 22, 2003.
17. For a review of the transmission of SARS on airlines, see "Consensus document on the epidemiology of severe acute respiratory syndrome (SARS)," Department of Communicable Disease Surveillance and Response, WHO, Geneva, 2003, http://www.who.int/csr/sars/en/WHOconsensus.pdf.
18. Ibid.
19. Stohr describes setting up the network and the ground rules for its operation in an article he published anonymously in the *Lancet*. "A multicentre collaboration to investigate the cause of severe acute respiratory syndrome," *Lancet* 2003, 361: 1730.
20. Personal interview.
21. See also Chapter 2.
22. Personal interview.
23. "New light shed on pneumonia outbreak," *China Daily*, March 20, 2003.
24. Brundtland interview, WHO SARS Oral History,
25. Ibid.
26. Yukifumi Takeuchi, "WHO chief: China too secretive at start of SARS outbreak," *Asahi Shimbun* April 9, 2003.
27. Brundtland interview, WHO SARS Oral History, June 2003
28. "Secretary Thompson, Chinese Minister Vow to Cooperate on SARS," United States Department of Health and Human Services News Release, April 4, 2003, http://www.hhs.gov/news.
29. Reported by Reuters news agency, April 17, 2003.
30. Speech by Premier Wen Jiabao at the Special China-ASEAN Leaders Meeting on SARS, April 29, 2004
31. WHO press release, July 5, 2003, http://www.who.int/mediacentre/releases/2003/pr56/en.
32. Ilona Kickbusch, "SARS: Wake-Up Call for a Strong Global Health Policy," *Yale Global Online*, April 25 2003. www.yaleglobal.yale.edu.
33. Cited in Rob Stein, "WHO Gets Wider Power to Fight Global Health Threats," *The Washington Post*, May 28, 2003.

CHAPTER 5

1. For a vivid account of the plague outbreak in Hong Kong in 1894 and the race between two biologists, Alexander Yersin and Shibasaburo Kitazabo, to discover the microbe causing the disease, see Edward Marriott, *The Plague Race: a Tale of Fear, Science and Heroism*, New York: Picador, 2002.
2. Eric CJ Class, Albert DME Osterhaus, Ruud van Beek et al, "Human

influenza A H5N1 virus related to a highly pathogenic avian influenza virus," *Lancet* 1998, 351: 472–477. For a chronology of the H5N1 crisis, see *South China Morning Post*, Jan 24, 1998, p. 4.

3. Personal interview.
4. Personal interview.
5. Personal interview.
6. Personal interview.
7. Personal interview.
8. Emails from the German researchers announcing their findings can be found on the ProMED bulletin board of the International Society of Infectious Diseases, March 18 and 19, 2003, http://www.promedmail.org archive no. 20030319.0688. See also WHO press release http://www.who.int/csr/don/2003_03_19/en.
9. Email from John Tam, Department of Microbiology, Faculty of Medicine, The Chinese University of Hong Kong, to the Pro-MED bulletin, March 19, 2003, http://www.promedmail.org, archive no. 20030319.0688.
10 . http://app.moh.gov.sg/new/new02.asp?id-1&mid=5500.
11. See "Canada Communicable Disease Report," April 15, 2003, http://www.hc-sc.gc.ca/pphb-dgspsp/publicat/ccdr-rmtc/03vol29/dr2908cb.html.
12. Personal interview
13. WHO press conference, Geneva, March 21, 2003, http://www.who.int/csr/sars/press_2003_03_21/en.
14. WHO SARS update No 6, March 21, 2003, http://www.who.int/csr/sars/archive/2003_03_21/en.
15. "A multicentre collaboration to investigate the cause of severe acute respiratory syndrome," *Lancet* 2003, 361: 1730–1733.
16. Ibid.
17. Robert Walgate, "Cause of SARS disputed," *The Scientist*, April 11, 2003, http://www.biomedcentral.com/news/20030416/04.
18. WHO press conference, Geneva, March 25, 2003, http://www.who.int/csr/sars/2003_03_25/en.
19. WHO press conference, Geneva, April 16, 2003. http://www.who.int/csr/sars/press_2003_04_16/en/
20 . Thijs Kuiken, Ron AM Fouchier, Martin Schutten et al. "Newly discovered coronavirus as the primary cause of severe acute respiratory disease syndrome," *Lancet* 2003, 362: 263–270.
21. See dia/pressrel/r030324.htm" http://www.cdc.gov/od/oc/media/pressrel/r030324.htm, and http://www.cdc.gov/od/oc/media/transcripts/t030324.htm.
22. WHO press conference, Geneva, April 11, 2003, http://www.who.int/csr/sars/press_2003_04_11/en.
23. JSM Peiris, ST Lai, LLM Poon et al, "Coronavirus as a possible cause of severe acute respiratory syndrome," *Lancet* 2003, 361: 1319–25. Published online April 8, 2003.

24. Thomas G Ksiazek, Dean Erdman, Cynthia Goldsmith et al, "A Novel Coronavirus Associated with Severe Acute Respiratory Syndrome," *New England Journal of Medicine.* Published at http://www.nejm.org, April 10, 2003. Christian Drosten, Stephan Gunther, Wolfgang Presier et al, 'Identification of a Novel Coronavirus in Patients with Severe Acute Respiratory Syndrome," *New England Journal of Medicine.* Published at http://www.nejm.org, April 10, 2003.

25. Personal interview

26. Personal interview.

27. Reported by Xinhua, Feb 18, 2003.

28. "Breakthrough in SARS m«5se," *China Daily* online, April 5, 2003, http://www1.chinadaily.com.cn/en/doc/2003–04/05/content_160897.htm.

29. Martin Enserink, 'China's missed chance," *Science* 2003, 301: 294–296.

30. "Chinese Scientists Defeated by SARS," *China Youth Daily*, English translation published in *People's Daily* online, June 9, 2003, http://english.peopledaily.com.cn/200306/09/eng20030609_117919.shtml.

31. Marco A Marra, Steven JM Jones, Caroline Astell et al, "The Genome sequence of the SARS-Associated Coronavirus," *Science* 2003, 300: 1399–1404.

32. Ibid.

33. Alexandre Batalin, "Atypical Pneumonia Virus has been created artificially," RIA Novosti news agency, April 10, 2003, http://news.softpedia.com/news/2/2003/April/3045.shtml.

34. See for example Richard D Fisher Jr, "SARS crisis: Don't rule out linkages to China's Biowarfare," *China Brief*, Vol 3 No 8, April 22, 2003, http://china.jamestown.org.

35. Chandra Wickramasinghe, Milton Wainright and Jayant Narlikar, "SARS, a clue to its origins?" *Lancet* 2003, 361: 1832.

36. Y Guan, BJ Zheng, YQ He et al, "Isolation and characterization of viruses related to the SARS coronavirus from animals in Southern China," *Sciencexpress*, Sep 4, 2003, http://www.sciencexpress.org.

37. D Yu, H Li, R Hu et al, "Prevalance of IgG Antibody to SARS-Associated Coronavirus in Animal Traders — Guangdong Province, China 2003," *Morbidity and Mortality Weekly Report,* Centre for Diseases Control and Prevention, Atlanta, 2003, 986–987.

38. Y Guan, BJ Zheng, YQ He et al, "Isolation and characterization of viruses related to the SARS coronavirus from animals in Southern China."

39. Personal interview.

40. John Stavrinides and David S Guttman, "Mosaic Evolution of the Severe Acute Respiratory Syndrome Coronavirus," *Journal of Virology* 2004, 78: 76–82.

41. Denise Normile and Ding Yimin, "Civets Back on China's Menu," *Science* 2003, 301: 1031.

42. Byron EE Martina, Bart L Haagmans, Thijs Kuiken et al, "SARS virus infection of cats and ferrets," *Nature* 2003, 425: 915.

CHAPTER **6**

1. One hypothesis is that it originated among British soldiers in France. See JS Oxford, "The so-called Great Spanish Influenza Pandemic of 1918 might have originated in France in 1916," *Philos Trans R Soc Lond B Biol Sci* 2001, 356: 1857–1859. Another hypothesis suggests that it started in an isolated part of the state of Kansas in the US in early 1918. Other hypotheses suggest it could have begun in China.

2. Cited in Gina Kolata, *Flu: The Story of the Great Influenza Pandemic of 1918 and the Search for the Virus that Caused It,* Farrar Strauss and Giroux: New York, 1999.

3. Quoted in "The American Experience: Influenza 1918," http://www.pbs.org/wgbh/amex/influenza/peopleevents/pandeAmerx90.html.

4. Cited in Kolata, *Flu: The Story of the Great Influenza Pandemic of 1918 and the Search for the Virus that Caused It.*

5. Quoted in "The American Experience: Influenza 1918."

6. Cited in http://www.spartacus.schoolnet.co uk/FWWinfluenzia.htm.

7. Rod Daniels, "In Search of an Enigma: the Spanish Lady," *Mill Hill Essays*, National Institute of Medical Research (UK), 1998, http://www.nimr.mrc.ac.uk/millhillessays/1998/influenza1918.htm.

8. Martin, Meltzer, Nancy J Cox and Keiji Fukuda, "The Economic Impact of Pandemic Influenza in the United States: Priorities for Intervention," *Emerging Infectious Diseases* 1997, 5: 659–671.

9. WHO, "Pandemic Preparedness," http://www.who.int/csr/disease/influenza/pandemic.html.

10. Gautam Naik, "Forget SARS: WHO Expert Says He Fears the Flu More," *Wall Street Journal*, May 29, 2003.

11. Kennedy F Shortridge, "Influenza — a continuing detective story," *Lancet* 1999, 354: S29.

12. Robert G Webster, "Influenza," *Emerging Viruses*, ed. Stephen S Morse, New York: Oxford University Press, 1993.

13. See Ann H Reid and Jeffrey K Taubenberger, "The origin of the 1918 pandemic influenza virus: a continuing dilemma," *Journal of General Virology* 2003, 84: 2285–2292.

14. Eric CJ Claas, Albert DME Osterhaus, Ruud van Beek et al, "Human influenza A H5N1 virus related to a highly pathogenic avian influenza virus," *Lancet* 1998, 351: 421–427.

15. KF Shortridge, JSM Peiris and Y Guan, "The new influenza pandemic: lessons from Hong Kong," *Journal of Applied Microbiology* 2003, 94: 70S–79S.

16. For details see "Human Cases of Avian Influenza A (H7N7) Infection, The Netherlands, 2003," Centre for Diseases Control and Prevention Atlanta, http://www.cdc.gov/ncidod/diseases/flu/H7N7facs.htm.

17. In Gautam Naik, op cit.

18. Kim Young-hoon, "Bird Flu's spread threatens poultry industry," *Joong Ang Daily*, Dec 12, 2003.

19. Richard J Webby and Robert G Webster, "Are We Ready for Pandemic Influenza?" *Science* 2003, 302: 1519–1522.

20. Speech to WHO global meeting on SARS, Kuala Lumpur, June 17, 2003, http://www.who.int/csr/sars/conference/june_2003/materials/presentations/brundtland/en.

21. See notes 2 and 3

22. This would also depend on which stage of the disease patients with a new flu virus would be at their most infectious. In the case of SARS, patients became infectious when they started displaying symptoms of the disease. They then went to hospitals and doctors for treatment, exposing the virus to medical staff when they were at their most infectious. This might not be the case for a new flu epidemic.

23. Marty Logan, "Flu Pandemic Plan a World Away from South's Preparations," *Inter Press Service*, Feb 13, 2004.

24. Ibid.

INDEX